History of Nursing

History of Nursing

Echoes of Compassion: Tracing Nursing's Legacy Through Time

Second Edition

TK Indrani BSc (N)

Ex-Assistant Lecturer
College of Nursing
Sri Ramachandra Medical College and Research Institute
Sri Ramachandra Deemed University
Chennai, Tamil Nadu, India

Jitika Royal

MSN (Mental Health Nursing)
RNRM BSc (H) Nursing
New Delhi, India

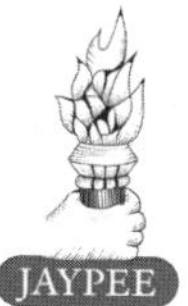

JAYPEE BROTHERS MEDICAL PUBLISHERS
The Health Sciences Publisher
New Delhi | London

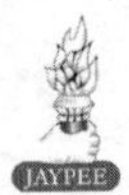

Jaypee Brothers Medical Publishers (P) Ltd

Headquarters
Jaypee Brothers Medical Publishers (P) Ltd
EMCA House, 23/23-B
Ansari Road, Daryaganj
New Delhi 110 002, India
Landline: +91-11-23272143, +91-11-23272703
+91-11-23282021, +91-11-23245672
Email: jaypee@jaypeebrothers.com

Corporate Office
Jaypee Brothers Medical Publishers (P) Ltd
4838/24, Ansari Road, Daryaganj
New Delhi 110 002, India
Phone: +91-11-43574357
Fax: +91-11-43574314
Email: jaypee@jaypeebrothers.com

Overseas Office
J.P. Medical Ltd
83 Victoria Street, London
SW1H 0HW (UK)
Phone: +44 20 3170 8910
Fax: +44 (0)20 3008 6180
Email: info@jpmedpub.com

Website: www.jaypeebrothers.com
Website: www.jaypeedigital.com

Inquiries for bulk sales may be solicited at: jaypee@jaypeebrothers.com

History of Nursing

First Edition: 2004

Second Edition: **2024**

ISBN: 978-93-5696-931-5

Printed in India at Sterling Graphics Pvt. Ltd.

The Nightingale's Pledge

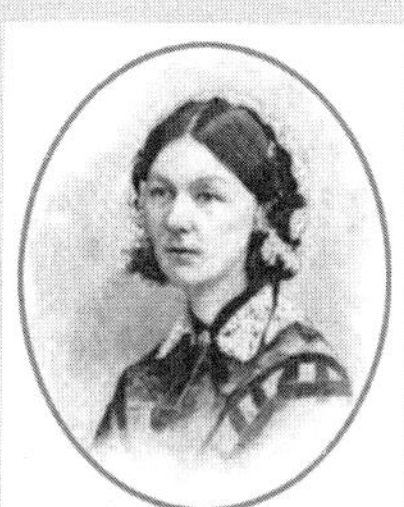

I solemnly pledge myself before God and in the presence of this assembly, to conscientiously practice my profession.

I will respect all life, dignity, rights of man in the practice of my calling.

I will zealously seek, to nurse those who need care irrespective of nationality, race, creed, color, age, sex, politics, or social status.

I will collaborate and coordinate, with health team, and devote myself to the welfare of my patients, my family, and my country.

I will endeavor to fulfill my rights and privileges as a good citizen, and take my share of responsibility to promote health, to prevent illness, to restore health, and to alleviate suffering.

I will constantly endeavor to increase my knowledge and skills in nursing, and to use them wisely.

I will be active in assisting others, in safeguarding and promoting the health, and happiness of mankind.

Preface to the Second Edition

Welcome to *History of Nursing* a comprehensive exploration of the evolution and impact of nursing throughout the ages. This book delves into the rich tapestry of nursing history, from its humble beginning to its current status as a vital profession in healthcare.

Through meticulous research and storytelling, We aim to shed light on the unsung heroes of nursing, whose dedication and compassion have shaped the field into what it is today. From Florence Nightingale to modern-day nursing pioneers, each chapter uncovers the challenges, triumphs, and innovations that have defined nursing practice.

Whether you are a seasoned healthcare professional, a student aspiring to join the ranks of nursing, or simply a curious reader interested in the history of this noble profession, *History of Nursing* offers a glimpse into the past that continues to inspire and inform the future of healthcare.

Thank you for embarking on this journey with us. We hope that this book serves as a tribute to the enduring legacy of nursing and the remarkable individuals who have dedicated their lives to caring for others.

TK Indrani
Jitika Royal

Preface to the First Edition

The title "History of Nursing" is an attempt by the author to define spectrum of nursing administration since its inception. Author has covered the chapters "Historical Developments in Nursing", nursing aspect and how different civilization felt about illness and what sort of nursing administration they were undertaking. All the developments in the field of nursing have been covered thoroughly. "What exactly the Modern Nursing is all about" has been duly dealt with. "The Scenario of Nursing in India" and "Continuing Education" are some of chapters where one can get the details they are looking for. The readers will find the book to be very helpful. All care has been taken to avoid errors to great extent.

TK Indrani

Acknowledgments

"The Lord Himself has given His Command; by His Grace, He has blessed me with His Glance of Grace."

—Sri Guru Granth Sahib Ji

First and foremost, we would like to thank Almighty Waheguru Ji. You have granted us strength to trust my passion and go after my aspirations.

We would like to express our sincere gratitude to all the individuals who have contributed to the creation of this book, *History of Nursing*.

We would also like to acknowledge the support and encouragement of our colleagues, friends, and family throughout the writing process. Your encouragement and feedback have been invaluable in bringing this project to fruition.

We owe thanks to M/s Jaypee Brothers Medical Publishers (P) Ltd, New Delhi, India especially we would like to express our gratitude to Shri Jitendar P Vij (Group Chairman), Mr Ankit Vij (Managing Director), Mr MS Mani (Group President), Dr Madhu Choudhary (Director-Educational Publishing), who are the continual source of inspiration throughout this journey. Ms Pooja Bhandari [Director-Production (Books and Journals)], Ms Sunita Katla (Executive Assistant to Group Chairman and Publishing Manager), Ms Samina Khan (Executive Assistant to Director-Educational Publishing), Mr Rajesh Sharma (Production Coordinator), Ms Seema Dogra (Cover Visualizer), Ms Neha Verma (Graphic Designer), Ms Geeta Barik (Proofreader), Mr Kulwant Singh (Typesetter) and Radhe Shyam (Graphic Designer) who added hue and life to the entire book and perfected the script.

Lastly, we extend our heartfelt thanks to the readers and enthusiasts of nursing history who continue to show interest and appreciation for the legacy and evolution of the nursing profession. Your passion for understanding the past informs and inspires the future of nursing practice.

Contents

Chapter 1: Historical Development in Nursing 1
- History of Nursing *2*
- Nursing in Early Civilizations *4*
- Early Christian Era *10*
- Early Middle Age *12*

Chapter 2: Contributions of Florence Nightingale 19

Chapter 3: Nursing in India 23
- Ancient History of Nursing in India *23*

Chapter 4: Nursing as a Profession 35
- Philosophy of Nursing *37*
- Scope of Nursing *45*

Chapter 5: Development of Nursing Education in India 49
- Evolution of Nursing Education in India *49*
- Nursing and Midwifery Council (NMC) *59*
- Ethical Aspects of Nursing *65*

Chapter 6: Code of Ethics 65
- Code of Ethics *65*

Chapter 7: Trends in Nursing 74
- Nursing Trends *74*

Chapter 8: Telemedicine and Telenursing 84
- Telemedicine in India *84*

Key Terms *95*

Index *99*

Chapter 1

Historical Development in Nursing

> *"The amount of relief and comfort experienced by the sick after the skin has been carefully washed and dried is one the commonest observations made at a sickbed."* ***—Florence Nightingale***

INTRODUCTION

Nursing, one of the oldest arts, remains an indispensable modern occupation rooted in the fundamental human need for care and comfort in times of illness and injury. Its origins can be traced back to the dawn of human existence, reflecting the intrinsic connection between nurturing and the preservation of life. The historical evidence underscores the crucial role of nursing in the very survival and development of the human race.

A comprehensive understanding of nursing's evolution requires delving into general history as a foundation to comprehend and interpret the dynamic changes that have shaped the profession. The roots of both medicine and nursing intricately weave through mythologies, ancient cultures in the East and West, and various religions.

Exploring the history of nursing enhances a nurse's awareness and fosters an appreciation of the social and intellectual foundations of the discipline. Since its inception, nursing has been a manifestation of community service dedicated to safeguarding and perpetuating the well-being of families. Notably, both men and women historically assumed nursing roles, highlighting the inclusive nature of the profession.

In ancient times, particularly during prehistoric periods, women played a pivotal role in gathering herbs, roots, and plants with medicinal properties, contributing to the healing of the sick. This early connection between women and herbal remedies laid the groundwork for the holistic approach that continues to characterize nursing today.

The symbiotic relationship between nursing and medicine has evolved over centuries, shaped by cultural, societal, and religious influences. Recognizing and appreciating this historical journey not only honors the profession but also informs contemporary nursing practices. As nursing continues to progress, acknowledging its rich history remains integral to cultivating a deep sense of purpose and dedication within the profession.

HISTORY OF NURSING

- Nursing has a rich history spanning centuries, predating its integration with modern medical practices.
- Within familial settings, the responsibility for nursing needs fell upon family members who attended to the sick at home.
- The advancement of medicine, surgery, and public health transformed into intricate technical domains, demanding specialized procedures performed by trained individuals with a deep understanding of scientific principles.
- This transformation gave rise to the nursing profession.
- Examining the historical trajectory of nursing reveals challenges faced in the past, the ingenious solutions found, and the rapid progress made despite hindrances.
- In early history, nursing emerged as a form of community service, rooted in the instinct to preserve and protect the family unit.
- Nursing originated from a fundamental desire to maintain health, extending care, comfort, and assurance to those in need.
- The history of nursing intricately weaves into the tapestry of healthcare, economic shifts, societal dynamics, and cultural trends.
- The profession's evolution mirrors and responds to these multifaceted influences.
- Ongoing transformations in healthcare are profoundly influencing the nursing profession.
- These contemporary changes underscore the dynamic nature of nursing and its adaptability to emerging challenges.

❖ In essence, nursing's enduring history, independent of modern medicine, reflects its intrinsic ties to family care and community service. The evolution of nursing as a profession resonates with the dynamic interplay of societal, cultural, and healthcare dynamics, with the profession continually adapting to meet evolving challenges.

Prehistoric Nursing

Myths, songs, and archaeological discoveries shed light on the prehistoric man's approach to caring for the sick. During this era, there was a prevailing belief that illnesses were caused by 'evil spirits infiltrating the body.' In response, various practices were employed to address the perceived intrusion of these malevolent forces. Prehistoric man believed that a thing in nature like tree or river had a spirit or soul.

The ill-treated body underwent harsh measures, including starvation, physical beatings, the administration of nauseous substances, drum beating, magical rites, ceremonies, and inducing sudden fright—all aimed at expelling the evil spirits believed to be responsible for the sickness. In this context, the figure serving as both a doctor and nurse was regarded as a magical practitioner, adept at wielding mystical forces to counteract and dispel the perceived malevolence causing illness. This multifaceted healer played a pivotal role in the prehistoric community's attempts to restore health and well-being by navigating the spiritual realm to counteract the perceived influences of evil spirits.

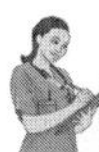

Role of Nurse in Primitive Period

The role of the nurse in primitive periods was characterized by women's maternal guardianship, providing basic healthcare to the family unit. Primitive nursing practices evolved to address the dual purpose of maintaining health and offering comfort, with a focus on caring, comforting, nourishing, and cleansing. Love and hope found expression in the empirical nursing practices of these early societies, emphasizing the foundational aspects of compassionate care which is shown in **Flowchart 1.1**.

Flowchart 1.1: Role of a nurse in primitive period.

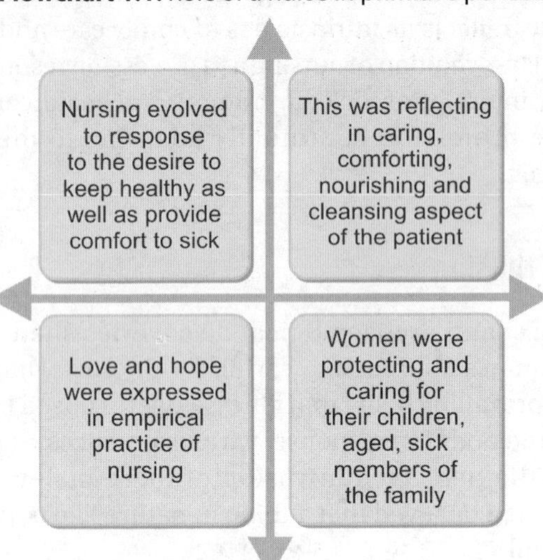

NURSING IN EARLY CIVILIZATIONS

The ancient cultures and practices of health care are depicted in **Figure 1.1**.

Sumerian

The Sumerians, who thrived around 5,000 years ago, were a fascinating ancient civilization. Rather than characterizing their religious practices as worshipping evil spirits, it's more accurate to say they had a polytheistic belief system, acknowledging a variety of deities. These Gods were associated with natural elements, societal concepts, and aspects of life.

Babylonias (New Iraq)

They believed, illness was caused by sun and anger by God. Temples became center for medical care. They brought the sick and obtained advice, diagnosis, and treatment of diseases. Their treatment consisted of giving better concoctions, in order to drive away the evil spirits from the rich persons. The team approach was used to treat the sick persons.

- Physician directed the treatment

Sumerians
Babylonias (New Iraq)
Persians (New Iran)
Ancient Egypt
Ancient Hebrews
Ancient Americans
Incas
Ancient India
Ancient China
Ancient Japan
Ancient Greek
Ancient Roman
Irish Cults

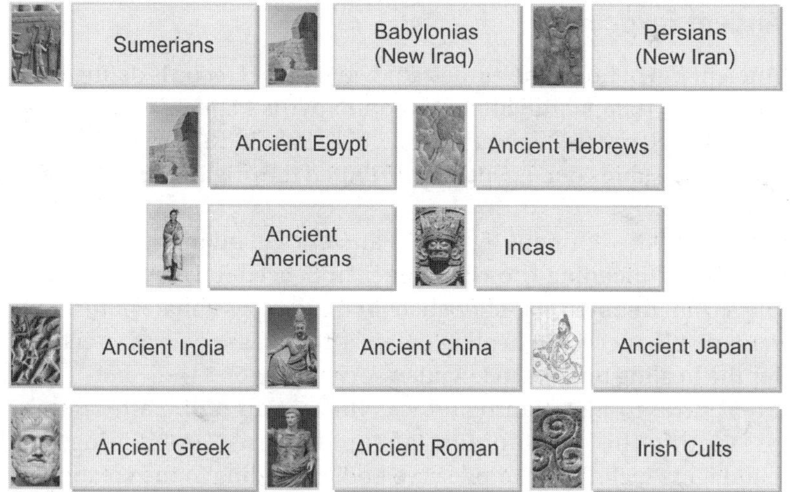

Fig 1.1: Types of ancient cultures.

- Nurse carried out the case
- The pharmacies prepared the medicine
- Along with this spiritual care was also given.
  So, the Babylonias believed that sin was the causes by anger of God.

Persians (New Iran)

Persians were a group of Iranian tribes. Their religion at the time was Zoaras Tronums founder of this was "Prophet Zoraster". The Parsees in India are descendants of the Persians. They believed in "evil spirit theory of disease". Their holy book is called *Avesta*. This describes ceremonial rules of laws for birth and death. After a person's death body was fastened to the roof of a special high tower called "Tower of silence". The birds picked the flesh, bones, dropped to the pit below the tower.

The Health Care

Three types of practitioners came out of their medical centers:
1. Those who heal with the knife
2. Those heal with herbs
3. Those with holy words

Ancient Egypt

Ancient Egypt holds the earliest known medical records dating back to around 1600 BC, documented on Papyrus Paper. Among these, the "Ebers Papyrus," famously brought to light in 1874 by Dr Ebers of Germany, stands out. Egyptians attributed the origins of medicine to divine sources.

One of the eminent figures in ancient Egyptian medicine was "Imhotep," meaning "he who comes in peace." Revered as a priest physician, Imhotep was cherished for his compassionate nature and remarkable success in healing the sick. Temples served as vital hubs for the healing process in Egyptian society.

Central to Egyptian belief was the notion of life after death, prompting the development of sophisticated embalming and bandaging techniques to preserve bodies, leading to the creation of mummies. These preserved bodies offer invaluable insights into the diseases and treatments of the time.

High-ranking women in Egyptian society often assumed roles as priestesses in temples, where some assisted in caring for the sick. Moreover, within households, mothers and daughters played significant roles in nursing the ill. Despite their advancements, Egyptians strictly prohibited the dissection of deceased bodies.

Ancient Hebrews

The best source book of the history of Hebrews, is the Old Testament of a Bible. Many rules and regulations in regard to social and religious customs, healthy, sanitary practices are compiled into, what is called the Mosaic code. This code presents, a systematic organized method of practice of disease. It includes principles of personal hygiene to rest, sleep, cleanliness, hours of works and special rules for women. Principles of public hygiene and sanitation regarding food, disposal waste of excrete and garbage, isolation, quarantine disinfection and reporting of communicable disease. Isolation keeping some diseased person separately, quarantine supporting the disease will be disappeared, we have tendencies to spread to others. So, they are kept separately, and reporting of communicable disease. The high priest was "priest physician" and health inspector. Houses of hospitality, forerunner of inns, hotel and hospital. They practized excellent hospitality, visiting and caring for the sick was religious duty. A nurses role includes a midwifery.

Ancient Americans

Before Columbus discovered America, a highly developed culture flourished there. There were many different groups, but much is known about Mayas, Eucas, AZTECS. The priest was the medical advisor and pharmacists. They practiced sweat bath. The AZTECS were war like group ruling central America. They also practiced sweat bath and human sacrifice to cure diseases.

Incas

Incas empire was located in Peru in America. They were skilled engineer at supervision bridges. They practiced "Trephin ring" (making hole in the skull to cure disease) and applied cranial bandage skills. They also believed diseases were caused by anger of God. Disease gift to the God were in the forms of "Effigy". The Incas also practiced "sand painting" to cure the disease.

Sand painting, applied to the sense of right. Prayerful singing to the sense of hearing the sweet-smelling herbs, to the sense of small, and the herbs to be eaten to the sense of taste, faith on the part of the patients. In addition to their technique, they also practiced "Hydrotherapy" (bringing down the temp down) into the healing ceremony.

Ancient China

The Chinese doctors used systematic methods of diagnosis like our modern doctor, the Chinese doctor's slogan was look, listen, ask and feel. Among the Chinese doctor "Sen lung was known as father of medicine in China and an authority of an internal medicine. The Chinese doctors practiced "vaccination" as earlier 1000 BC. They used "seaweed" to cause thyroid conditions and chaul mogra oil for curing leprosy. As earlier as 13,000 AD physiotherapy was also used, as part of treatment. They recognized disease such as "Syphilis and Gonorrhea". They also had halls, near to temple where the sick prayed for healing hygiene was important, bathing and wearing clothes were advised and practiced. Tea drinking was an ancient precaution in China, against intestinal infections. The Chinese believed when disease due to the evil spirits in the patients. Thus, nursing was impossible, and this faith also prevented the progress of medical progress.

Ancient Japan

Japanese copied Chinese system of medicine. They developed the art of acupuncture. Today, it is a highly specialized branch of medicine, practiced all over the world.

Ancient India

3000 BC

The Ayurvedic system placed significant emphasis on promoting hygiene, preventing sickness, and implementing measures such as inoculation against smallpox. The importance of sanitation, proper ventilation, and well-equipped kitchens was recognized. Hospitals were constructed, and efforts were made to cultivate medicinal plants. Additionally, suitable accommodations were provided for animals.

600–700 BC

Nursing played a crucial role in patient care. Nurses were described as cool-headed and pleasant, refraining from speaking ill of others. They were strong, attentive to the needs of the sick, and diligently followed physicians' instructions. According to Charakha Sanhita, nursing attendants were expected to be resourceful, devoted, and possess purity of mind and body. Good behavior, along with distinguished cleanliness habits, was deemed essential. Nursing treatments included baths, enemas, emetics, infusions, venesection, gargles, massages, and limb manipulation. Nurses assisted patients in movement and bed-making, while also being skilled in compounding drugs.

226–250 BC

King Ashoka made significant contributions by constructing monasteries and hospitals for both humans and animals. Physicians and midwives were required to be trustworthy and skilful, adhering to cleanliness standards. Surgical procedures were preceded by religious ceremonies and prayers. Interestingly, nursing attendants were predominantly men or elderly women. Women took care of sick family members, showcasing a dedication to patient well-being, despite the often-unrewarded nature of their work. Desirable qualities for nursing attendants included good behavior, purity, kindness, and skill.

Recognizing the importance of nursing, King Ashoka implemented provisions for the education and training of women for this purpose.

Ancient Greek

The early Greeks believed in medicine of divine origin and was represented by many Gods, e.g., Apollo, the sun God, the God of health and medicine. Asklepios, the God of healing, Hygenia, the Goddess of health. Temples were built for these Gods. People come here, not only to worship the God, but also to get treatment for illness or disease. Incubation was practiced during illness. Medical treatments included special diets, massage, bath, "Inunciation" (rubbing medicine on skin). The uncleaned patients like delivered lady and dying patients were not allowed to come in the temple or remain throughout. In 1070 AD special buildings were erected for their patients. They were regarded as the first "Europeon hospitals".

Hippocrates

Hippocrates, revered as the Father of Medicine, was born Circa 460 BC. Through meticulous observation of symptoms, he dispelled the notion that diseases stemmed from malevolent spirits, attributing them instead to humanity's disregard for natural laws.

The prevention of diseases, according to Hippocrates, hinged upon obedience to the laws of nature, marking the dawn of scientific medicine. He pioneered methods for conducting physical examinations and obtaining medical histories. Emphasizing the importance of fresh air, cleanliness, and a nutritious diet, he laid the foundation for holistic health practices.

Hippocrates provided guidance on various treatments, including hot applications, poultices, and cold sponging for fever. He also advocated for fluids in managing kidney diseases and mouthwashes for oral health.

Central to Hippocrates' teachings was the concept of professional integrity and accountability, reflected in the enduring "Hippocratic Oath" still administered in medical schools today.

The Caduces

Insignia of medical profession is one of the gifts from Greeks, i.e., symbol is associated with "AESCULA PEUS" of Greek mythology. The

"The CADUCEUS" is one of the gifts from Greek. It is composed of the staff intewined with serpents. This staff indicates the traveler, the intertwined serpents signify Rejuvenated, knowledge and wisdom. The Epics (tip) of the staff, are two wings of mercury (God of Greek) for speed, with which a physician should act.

Ancient Roman

Romans copied much from Greeks (system of medicine). Many physicians were Greek slave, who did not believe in Roman superstition. The early hospitals in Roman were built for soldiers and slaves, old women and men of good character did the nursing. In the ruins of Poempeis. Many instruments, similar to our modern surgical, scalpel, forceps speculum were found.

Irish Cults (Ireland was Called "Hibernia")

Many of these, Irish people were migrated of non-Europe and brought with them the richness of art, music and literature. They practised moist, heat in treatment, believed attending to the peace of mind and patients.

EARLY CHRISTIAN ERA

1–500 AD

1 AD to 500 AD Pre-Christian times was influenced by various religious beliefs they accepted diseases as punishment. Jesus Christ brought a new aspect that of Altruism (thoughtful interest in others). Christianity thought that kindly service to humanity, without any hope or reward. Followers of Jesus Christ took upon themselves the care of sick and poor. From early Christian Era, we have a continuous record of history of Nursing.

Apostolic Orders of Women

The church thought equality in men and women—assisted the clergy in the work of church. In the time, three were orders of women developed.

1. Deaconesses (those who are doing religious teachings)
2. A second order of widows
3. The virgin

Deaconesses

- Deaconesses did teachings and preachings and cared for their sick in their homes.
- A second order of widows also assisted—deaconesses with home visiting.
- The virgin are the younger women, assisted in caring for the Church Testaments and giving out alms to poor.
- One of the outstanding early deaconesses was Phoebe.
- Phoebe is known as the forerunner of modern public health nurse.
- The deaconesses order, disappeared after 4th century. Widows and virgins interested in religious works went to monasteries as nuns.

Widows

They assisted deaconess in home visiting. Freedom from responsibilities at home was a necessity.

Virgins

They were younger women, assisted in caring for church vestments and in giving alms to poor. They lived in their own homes and received no pay except when necessary. Order of virgins was created when church felt that virginity was essential to purity of life.

Xenodochia

As time went on Jesus was prosecuted. Many who were poor, sick turn to the Bishop of the Church for help. The Bishop home was too small to meet the demands of hospitality. So additional rooms and shelter were added. This was called xenodochia. In this all types of relief work were carried out, e.g., hospitals for the sick those with leprosy, home for strangers and orphans, aged and the travelers.

Roman Matrons

In Rome, women of high rank, had much freedom. As Christians they become interested, in works of charity and nursing. Some of the wealthy women formed an organized group used their wealth to found monasteries and hospitals. The well known among them was Marcella, Fabiola, Paula.

Marcella

She was the leader of this group. She had palace in best part of the Rome. She turned it into a Monastery. This was the first monastery in Rome.

Fabiola

Under the influence of Marcella, Fabiola become a Christian. She made a public confession of her sins and gave her wealth and energies for the care of the sick and poor. She turned her home into the first free Christian Hospital in Rome. She gathered the sicks from the streets and devoted her life to giving them nursing care.

Paula

Paula was a friend of Fabiola. She was wealthy and very intelligent. When her husband died she entered Marcella's monastery and there she became a Christian. About 385 AD, she and her daughter, Eustochia, went to Palestine and settled in Bethlehem. Here she built hospices (place of shelter for travelers) and hospitals for the sick. She and her staff did the nursing. She established a monastery in Bethlehem and gathered a group of devoted women. After her death, in 404 AD her work was carried on by her daughter.

EARLY MIDDLE AGE

Early middle age is a dark age in the history of nursing. This era began with the fall of the mighty Roman Empire. Barbonic tribes invaded Rome in 476 AD and brought about the final disorganization of society. During, this time, the Roman armies were disbanded. Roads and bridges were destroyed. "Roter hands" crowded the highways, making travel unsafe. People's homes were destroyed or taken over by the Barbarians turning many homeless.

Roman authorities shifted the capital from Rome to Constantinople. Due to this change in the capital, many of the aristocracy left for constantinople. Many of those who have to remain, turned to the Monasteries for help and protection. According to the self needs of the time. Three protectives units developed:

1. The Monasticism
2. The Feudalism and Chivalry
3. The Guilds

Monasticism

Monasticism means life, rules, conditions of monasteries. Monasteries where priests or nuns lived. The monasteries increased in size and facilities and new rules were set up to meet the needs of changing society. As time went on, many of the monks and nuns proved themselves to be exceptionally good organizers and administrators. One outstanding monk was St. Benedict of Nursia. He encouraged all his neighbors whether Pagan or Barbarians, to become Christians and to work together in harmony. He also built a monastery on a rocky mountain top between Rome and Naples called Monte Casino. Monte Casino grew to become one of the most efficient medieval monasteries. Here the Benedictine rule was developed to meet their needs. In addition to customary monastic vows of poverty, chastity and obedience vow of lifelong service was made. Men and women were allowed to live purposeful lives devoted to the kind of work they enjoyed. Men and women from all ranks and social classes were admitted to the Benedictine order. It became one of the most active organizations for social work.

Feudalism and Chivalry

Following the fall of Rome, much of the agricultural land was controlled by a class of gentlemen farmers. The homeless turned to these landlords for protection. Thus, an ancient system known as feudalism, but modified by Christian ideals came into existence along with monasticism. In feudalism the king owned all the land. He gave portions of the land to his favorite subjects who were barons, earls, or knights. These grants of land were known as a fief or feud in Europe and a manor in England. The Baron divided his land among many serfs who worked on the land in return for food, shelter, and a form of protection. Since, there was no standing army the landlord might call on the serfs to leave the land and serve in his army when necessary. The serf had very little freedom. If the land was sold, he became the serf of the new owner. Petty quarrels among the knight took place and kept the serfs from the land. This resulted in famine and disease. The training of the knight, which become known as **"chivalry'** stressed service to others, protection and defense of the weak. Every true knight came to believe that service to God came before service to his earthly lord, chivalry was the accepted code for living a good life.

Guilds

This was the first organization of workmen and tradesmen who were not attached to monastic or feudal groups. Divided into three categories these guilds protected the worker, the products and the public. In the guilds apprenticeship method of learning a skill was stressed higher standards of work encouraged, unethical practices were checked and social insurances including sickness. Insurances were followed. This guild apprenticeship method has been followed in nursing and medical teaching for many years. Also, the guild was the forerunner of the modern labor unions and professional organizations.

Special Care of Mentally Ill

The first organized plan for the care of mentally ill and retarted children was found in Greece, Belgium. St Dymphma had been made the Patron saint of mentally ill people.

Medieval Hospitals

There were three famous medieval hospitals built outside monastery walls which are still in existence.

1. Hotel—Dieu of fyons in France
2. The Hostel Dieu of Paris
3. The Saints Spirito Hospital of the Holy Ghost in Rome

British Period (16th Century Onwards)

After the Mughal period the nursing in India hindered due to various reasons like low state of women, system of "Pardha" among Muslims, caste system among Hindus, illiteracy, poverty, political unrest, language difference and nursing looked upon as servants work. During the 16th century, nursing development in India taken three dimensions:

1. Military Nursing
2. Civilian Nursing
3. Missionaries Nursing

History of Military Nursing in India

Military nursing emerged during the First World War but saw gradual development thereafter. Recognizing the need for nursing care for

British officials and soldiers in India, British officers called for action. On February 21, 1888, ten fully qualified certified nurses trained by Florence Nightingale arrived in Mumbai, laying the groundwork for nursing in India and paving the way for its eventual excellence.

In 1894, a regular training system for men in hospital work, specifically as orderlies, was initiated. Some men volunteered for the course, seeking nursing certificates. Following two months of practical ward experience and supervised reports from senior sisters, the first official hospital orderly certificates were issued, establishing the foundation for future training and education systems.

In 1927, the Indian Military Nursing Services was formally described, comprising 12 matrons, 18 sisters, and 25 staff nurses. They were entrusted with supervising, instructing, and training nursing services for the entire Indian hospital corps.

During the Second World War, nursing services expanded both in India and overseas under the direction of the chief principal matron. A three-year training program was established in selected military hospital preliminary training schools. Upon successful completion, nurses were awarded certificates as "Registered Nurses" and became members of the Indian Military Nursing Services, Auxiliary Nursing Services.

Facing a shortage of trained nurses in India after the Second World War, the government initiated a short, intensive training course in 1942, leading to the establishment of the Auxiliary Nursing Services. Basic training for six months was conducted in selected civil hospitals. Following examinations at military hospitals in India, trainees were sent overseas to serve as 'Assistant Nurses', with 3,000 women undergoing auxiliary training.

Civilian Nursing in India

- In 1664, the East India Company constructed the Government General Hospital in Chennai to serve civilians. By 1871, this hospital had taken on the responsibility of training nurses.
- In the mid-1850s, a training school for midwives was established, granting certificates of 'Diploma in Midwifery' to successful students and 'sick nursing' to those who did not pass. For the first time, six nurses graduated with the Diploma in Midwifery, marking a significant milestone in nursing education.

Missionary Nursing in India

Missionary nursing initiatives commenced training programs for Indian individuals to become nurses, with support from various countries. This led to the emergence of fully qualified Indian nurses. However, numerous obstacles hindered the development of nursing during those times:

- Girls faced restrictions on engaging in work.
- People held degrading and unworthy attitudes towards nursing.
- Hindus encountered obstacles due to the entrenched caste system.
- Muslims were marginalized under the 'pardah' system.

To address these challenges, Christian girls were initially encouraged and trained in nursing. Despite frequent disappointments and difficulties, nursing training gradually took shape. Initially, there was a lack of uniformity in nursing education, with no specific standards in place. However, from 1888 to 1893, a collaborative effort involving experts such as doctors, surgeons, nursing superintendents, and pharmacists resulted in the development of a curriculum for nursing training.

Between 1907 and 1910, the North India United Board of Examiners was established to oversee nursing administration and maintain standards. In 1928, a Hindi textbook for nurses was developed, further enhancing nursing education. Additionally, in 1939, efforts were made to establish postgraduate schools for nurses, marking significant progress in the field of nursing education and professional development.

Community Health Nursing

Community health nursing (CHN) gained traction with the formation of the Visiting Nurses Association by William Rathbone in England. This initiative emphasized charity and free care. Florence Lees further enhanced the Visiting Nurses program by providing specialized training for their work. This model influenced India due to the dire conditions under which children were being born, leading to high mortality rates. Untrained 'Dais' was attending to women during childbirth, unwilling to undergo training, and patients were often hesitant to accept new methods.

In response to this situation, the Midwives Registration Act was passed in 1926 to improve the training of midwives. Recognizing the need for community nursing training, the government gradually began to address this issue. In 1946, CHN was integrated into the Basic Nursing Program at institutions such as Delhi, Vellore, and Chennai, marking a significant step towards addressing the healthcare needs of communities in India.

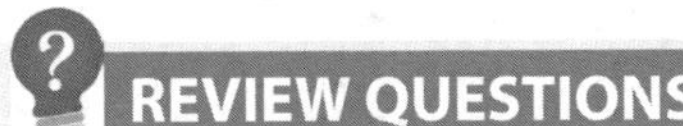

The historical development of nursing can be traced back to ancient civilizations, where care for the sick and injured was provided by family members or religious figures. Over time, nursing evolved into a formal profession with the establishment of religious orders dedicated to caring for the sick. In the 19th century, pioneers like Florence Nightingale revolutionized nursing by emphasizing hygiene, patient care, and education. The establishment of nursing schools and professional organizations further solidified nursing as a respected profession. Today, nursing continues to evolve with advancements in technology, research, and education, shaping the future of healthcare

REVIEW QUESTIONS

Long Answer Question

1. Write in detail about the historical development of nursing.

Short Answer Question

1. Explain the role of nurse in primitive period.

Multiple Choice Questions

1. Which ancient civilization is known for its early development of nursing practices and the establishment of temples dedicated to healing?
   A. Ancient Greece B. Ancient Egypt
   C. Mesopotamia D. Ancient China

Ans: B. Ancient Egypt

Explanation: Ancient Egypt is renowned for its advanced medical practices, including nursing. Temples dedicated to the God Imhotep, who was considered the patron of healing, served as centers for medical care and education, where priests and priestesses practiced various medical procedures, including nursing.

2. In which year the East India Company constructed the Government General Hospital in Chennai to serve civilians?
   A. 1928 B. 1939
   C. 1664 D. 1871

Ans: C. 1664

Explanation: In 1664, the East India Company constructed the Government General Hospital in Chennai to serve civilians. By 1871, this hospital had taken on the responsibility of training nurses.

3. In which year Community Health Nursing was integrated into the Basic Nursing Program at institutions in Delhi?

   A. 1926 B. 1936

   C. 1946 D. 1956

Ans: C. 1946

Explanation: In 1946, Community Health Nursing was integrated into the Basic Nursing Program at institutions such as Delhi, Vellore, and Chennai, marking a significant step towards addressing the healthcare needs of communities in India.

Chapter 2

Contributions of Florence Nightingale

"Quality is not an act; it is a habit." —***Aristotle***

INTRODUCTION

Florence Nightingale is renowned as the pioneer of modern nursing in 19th century. Born on May 12, 1820, in Florence, Italy, she was named after the city of her birth. As the second daughter of a prominent and wealthy British family, Florence demonstrated a deep commitment to serving others from a young age. During her teenage years, she dedicated her time to assisting the sick and impoverished in the village near her family estate, firmly believing that nursing was her vocation.

Despite her affluent background, Florence faced resistance from her parents when she declared her intention to pursue a nursing career. Undeterred by their disapproval, she defied societal norms and embarked on her nursing journey. In 1850, she enrolled as a nursing student at the Kaiserwerth Deaconesses' Institute in Düsseldorf, Germany, where she underwent four months of rigorous training.

Nightingale's work make her popular with the men. They called her "The Lady of the Lamp", **(Fig. 2.1)** in recognition of her Turkish candle lantern, which she carried through the corridors packed with wounded soldiers. After returning back to England after war, she established a teaching institution for nurses at St Thomas Hospital and at King's College Hospital in London. Within a few years after its foundation, the Nightingale School began receiving requests for nurses to found new schools and hospitals worldwide and Nightingale's reputation as the founder of modern nursing was assured. During her career, Nightingale concentrated on army sanitation reform, army hospitals and sanitation in India and among the poorer classed in England. For her efforts, Nightingale received numerous honors, including the

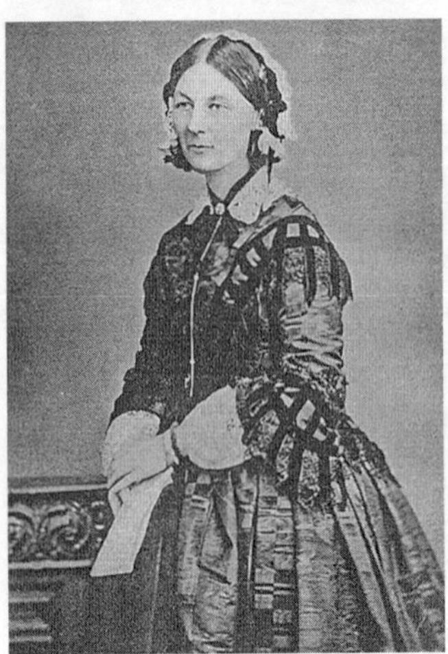

Fig. 2.1: Florence Nightingale (lady with the lamp).

Order of Merit from King Edward VII, Germany's Cross of Merit and France's Secours Aux Blesses Militaries. She wrote between 15,000 and 20,000 letters to friends and distinguished acquaintances. Nightingale was regarded as pioneer in the graphic display of statistics and was elected as the fellow of the Royal Statistical Society in 1858. In 1874, an honorary membership in the American Statistical Association was bestowed on her. Her writings, Notes on Matters Affecting the Health, Efficiency and Hospital Administration of the British Army (1858), Notes on Hospitals (1858), Notes on Nursing (1859), Notes on the Sanitary States of the Army in India (1871), and Life or Death in India (1874), reflect her continuing concerns about these issues. She worked into her eighties gathering data about nursing and healthcare. She died in her sleep at the age of 90 on August 13, 1910 in London.

She made significant contributions to healthcare and public health. Here are some of her key contributions:

- **Founder of modern nursing:** Florence Nightingale is often regarded as the founder of modern nursing. She transformed nursing into a respected and trained profession. Her work during the Crimean War (1853–1856) demonstrated the importance of sanitation, hygiene, and basic medical care in improving patient outcomes.

- **Nursing education:** Nightingale advocated for formal education and training for nurses. She established the Nightingale Training School for Nurses at St. Thomas' Hospital in London in 1860, laying the foundation for professional nursing education.
- **Statistical analysis and epidemiology:** Nightingale was a pioneer in the use of statistical analysis in healthcare. She collected and analyzed data to demonstrate the significance of sanitary conditions in preventing diseases. Her use of statistical charts and graphs helped to illustrate the impact of clean water, ventilation, and proper sanitation on reducing mortality rates.
- **Sanitary reforms:** Based on her observations and research, Nightingale emphasized the importance of maintaining clean and sanitary conditions in hospitals. She advocated for proper ventilation, clean water supply, and waste disposal to prevent the spread of infections.
- **Advocacy for public health:** Beyond her work in nursing, Nightingale was a vocal advocate for public health. She worked to improve living conditions in impoverished areas and campaigned for better sanitation and healthcare for all.
- **Writing and literature:** Nightingale was a prolific writer, and her books and publications had a profound impact on healthcare practices. Her most famous work, "Notes on Nursing: What It Is and What It Is Not," provided practical guidance for nurses and laid the groundwork for nursing as a profession.
- **International influence:** Nightingale's influence extended beyond the United Kingdom. Her ideas and principles had a global impact on nursing education, healthcare reform, and public health practices.
- **Legacy in nursing:** Florence Nightingale's legacy continues in the form of the Florence Nightingale Pledge, a modified version of the Hippocratic Oath taken by nurses. Nurses around the world still honor her contributions and commitment to compassionate care.

Florence Nightingale's contributions significantly shaped the nursing profession, revolutionized healthcare practices, and laid the groundwork for modern public health initiatives. Her work continues to inspire and influence healthcare professionals today.

SUMMARY

Florence Nightingale, known as the founder of modern nursing, made significant contributions to the field of healthcare. She is best known for her work during the Crimean War, where she and her team of nurses improved sanitation and medical care in military hospitals, reducing the mortality rate significantly. Nightingale's emphasis on hygiene, patient care, and data-driven decision-making revolutionized nursing practices. She also played a key role in establishing nursing as a respected profession by advocating for education and training for nurses. Nightingale's legacy continues to inspire nurses worldwide to provide compassionate and evidence-based care to patients.

REVIEW QUESTIONS

Long Answer Question

1. Write in detail about the history of Florence Nightingale.

Short Answer Question

1. Write about the contribution of Florence nightingale in the field of nursing.

Multiple Choice Questions

1. Who is considered the founder of modern nursing?
   A. Clara Barton B. Florence Nightingale
   C. Mary Seacole D. Dorothea Dix

Ans: B. Florence Nightingale

Explanation: Florence Nightingale is widely regarded as the founder of modern nursing due to her pioneering work during the Crimean War and her contributions to nursing education, practice, and healthcare reform.

2. Who is known as the "Lady with the Lamp" and is considered the founder of modern nursing?
   A. Clara Barton B. Florence Nightingale
   C. Mary Seacole D. Dorothea Dix

Ans: B. Florence Nightingale

Explanation: Florence Nightingale earned the nickname "Lady with the Lamp" for her compassionate care of wounded soldiers during the Crimean War and is widely regarded as the founder of modern nursing due to her pioneering work and significant contributions to the field.

3. In which century did modern nursing as a profession emerge?
   A. 17th century B. 18th century
   C. 19th century D. 20th century

Ans: C. 19th century

Explanation: Modern nursing emerged as a profession in the 19th century, with notable figures like Florence Nightingale making significant contributions to its development during this time period.

Chapter 3

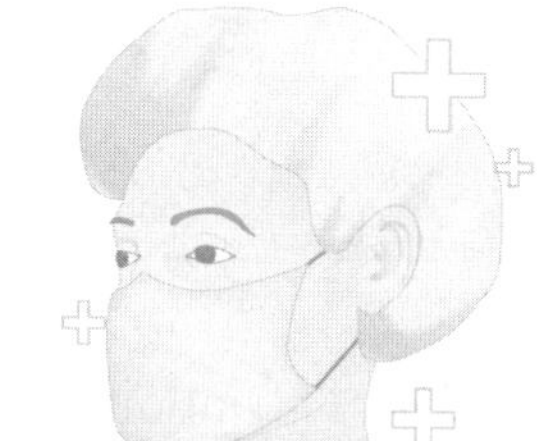

Nursing in India

> *"To succeed in your mission, you must have single-minded devotion to your goal."*
> ***—APJ Abdul Kalam***

INTRODUCTION

Nursing in India has a rich history that predates the modern era of medicine. Traditionally, within families, members provided care for the sick, meeting their nursing needs. Over time, the evolution of medicine, surgery, and public health transformed these practices into complex technical fields requiring specialized training and a deep understanding of scientific principles. This transformation brought nursing closer to modern medicine, bridging the gap between the two professions.

Historically, nursing in India has ancient roots. Before the 20th century, nursing practices were often carried out by young men, while women primarily served as midwives, assisting with childbirth. However, the landscape of nursing has significantly evolved since then.

Today, nursing in India has seen substantial improvements, particularly in the quality of education and clinical exposure provided to students. This enhanced education equips nurses with the necessary knowledge and skills to provide high-quality care to patients, families, and communities across the nation. By integrating modern medical advancements with traditional nursing principles, the profession continues to advance, ensuring better health outcomes and an improved quality of life for all.

ANCIENT HISTORY OF NURSING IN INDIA

- The ancient history of nursing in India reflects a longstanding tradition of providing care for the medical needs of individuals within the nation. This historical narrative underscores the antiquity of nursing principles and practices in the region.

- Formal nursing education began to take shape in the late 19th century. Notably, the inaugural nursing program was established at the Government General Hospital in Chennai, offering a six-month diploma course in midwifery to four students in 1871. Dr Alice Marval furthered this initiative by inaugurating the first nursing school for women at Saint Catherine's Hospital in Kanpur.
- During this period, efforts were made to enhance nursing standards by recruiting four female superintendents and four trained nurses from England to serve in Chennai. Between 1890 and 1900, numerous nursing schools were founded across India, facilitated by both missionary endeavors and government support. Additionally, the 20th century saw the establishment of national nursing associations, furthering the professionalization of the field.
- In 1897, BC Roy played a significant role in advocating for improved nursing standards and recognizing the contributions of nurses from both genders.
- The ancient practices of nursing in India are strikingly clear and resonate with modern nursing textbooks, highlighting the enduring nature of these caregiving traditions. Prior to the 20th century, nursing in India predominantly involved young men, while women primarily served as midwives assisting with childbirth.
- However, the acceptance of nursing as a profession in India encountered obstacles rooted in societal factors such as the low status of women, the caste system, illiteracy, and political unrest. It wasn't until the 17th century that formal exploration of nursing began, with each village typically having a midwife or traditional birth attendant to address maternal and child health needs.

In summary, while the formalization of nursing education and professional standards is relatively recent, the ancient history of nursing in India showcases a deep-rooted tradition of caregiving that has evolved over centuries to meet the healthcare needs of the population.

Nursing in Prehistoric Times

- The historical evidence regarding nursing care in prehistoric times is scarce, often inferred from myths, songs, and archaeological findings. Primitive societies employed various methods, including rituals to dispel evil spirits, such as beating, starvation, magical rites, nauseating medicines, loud noises, and sudden fright. Despite these practices, primitive individuals possessed rudimentary medical skills, such as massaging, fermentation, bone setting, amputation, and the application of hot and cold baths to control hemorrhages.

- In the primitive period, women played a significant role in nursing, tending to the needs of children, the elderly, and the sick within their families. Nursing practices evolved as a response to the innate human desire to maintain health and provide comfort to the ill. This nurturing instinct manifested in actions such as caring, comforting, nourishing, and cleansing the patient. These acts of love and hope were expressed through empirical nursing practices, reflecting an early understanding of the importance of compassionate care in promoting well-being and recovery.

Nursing-Vedic Period (3000–1400 BC)

During the Vedic period (3000–1400 BC) in India, ancient medical knowledge was documented in the sacred texts known as the "Vedas." It is believed that the principles of Ayurveda, the traditional system of medicine, were bestowed by Brahma during this time.

In 1400 BC, Sushruta, often referred to as the 'Father of Surgery' in India, authored a seminal text on surgery. Subsequently, Charaka composed a comprehensive treatise on internal medicine. These writings provide valuable insights into the advanced state of surgical practices during this era, which included the concept of 'Chatushpada Chikitsa,' comprising four essential components:

1. Physician (Bhishak)
2. Nurse (Upacharika or Attendant - Anuraktha)
3. Therapeutic drugs (Dravya)
4. Patient (Adhyaya)

The role of the nurse, referred to as Upacharika or Attendant, was characterized by several attributes:

- **Shuchi:** The nurse was expected to maintain purity and cleanliness both physically and mentally.
- **Daksha:** Competency was essential, indicating proficiency and skill in caregiving duties.

- **Anuraktha:** The nurse was required to demonstrate willingness and dedication in providing care and support to the patient.
- **Buddhiman:** Intelligence and effective communication skills were crucial for the nurse to act as a liaison between the patient and the physician, ensuring seamless coordination of care.

Nursing Post Vedic Period (600 BC–600 AD)

- Medical education flourished in the ancient universities of Nalanda and Taxila, where scholars from various disciplines congregated to pursue knowledge. During the reign of King Ashoka (272–236 BC), hospitals were established for the welfare of both people and animals, reflecting a commitment to healthcare across the realm.
- Prevention of diseases was prioritized during this period, with a strong emphasis on adopting hygienic practices. Cleanliness was considered a religious duty, with medical practitioners, including doctors and midwives, expected to be trustworthy and skilled. They were required to maintain personal hygiene by wearing clean clothes and keeping their nails short.
- Lying rooms in hospitals were meticulously maintained with proper ventilation to ensure a healthy environment for patients. Moreover, medical procedures were often preceded by religious ceremonies and prayers, underscoring the spiritual significance attributed to healing practices during ancient times. These rituals not only provided solace to patients but also fostered a sense of cooperation and harmony within the community.
- During the 1st century AD period, nursing was primarily carried out by men or elderly women in ancient societies. Women often faced restrictions on their activities outside the home but played a crucial role in caring for sick family members within domestic settings. However, superstitions and beliefs in black magic became prevalent during this time, sometimes overshadowing more practical caregiving practices.
- Medical knowledge and the administration of medicines were largely controlled by priest-physicians, who often refrained from handling blood and pathological tissues due to religious beliefs. Additionally, dissection was forbidden, and other religious restrictions and superstitious practices may have hindered the development of nursing during this period.

Nursing in Mughal Period (1000 AD)

- During the Mughal period (1000 AD), the practice of nursing in the Indo-Pakistani subcontinent was influenced by the development of the Unani system of medicine, which originated during the Arab civilization. This system of medicine, practiced widely in the region, is based on the concept of the four humors: blood, phlegm, yellow bile, and black bile. According to Unani principles, the temperament, strength, and natural balance of the body are central to maintaining health and treating illness.
- Unlike some other medical systems, Unani does not solely focus on eradicating diseases but emphasizes strengthening the body's defense mechanisms and promoting self-care and positive health habits. As a result, Unani medicine became an integral part of healthcare practices in the Indian subcontinent during the Mughal period.
- In the realm of nursing, practitioners would have drawn upon Unani principles to provide care that aimed to restore balance and harmony within the body, often through natural remedies, dietary adjustments, and lifestyle modifications. The emphasis on holistic health and preventive measures would have influenced nursing practices during this period, highlighting the importance of promoting overall well-being alongside the treatment of specific ailments.

Military Nursing in India

- Military nursing holds a significant place in the history of nursing, dating back to early centuries. One notable instance occurred in 1664 when the East India Company played a pivotal role in establishing a hospital for soldiers at Fort St. George in Chennai. Subsequently, a civilian hospital was erected, and medical personnel appointed by the East India Company served in both military and civilian medical facilities.
- The progression of military healthcare continued with the establishment of a Lying-in Hospital in 1797 and the government's authorization of a training school for midwives in 1894.
- However, one of the most notable advancements in military healthcare occurred in 1861, thanks to the pioneering efforts

of Miss Nightingale. Her advocacy and reforms within military hospitals not only transformed the quality of care for soldiers but also sparked reforms in civilian healthcare institutions.

- This highlights the enduring influence of military nursing on healthcare practices, as innovations and improvements made in military settings often transcend to benefit civilian healthcare systems as well.

Civilian Nursing in India

- In 1664, the East India Company established the Government General Hospital in Chennai to cater to civilian healthcare needs.
- By 1871, this hospital initiated the training of nurses, marking the formal beginning of nursing education in India.
- In 1854, a midwifery training school began granting certificates for "Diploma in Midwifery" to successful students and "sick nursing" to those who did not pass. Notably, this period saw the emergence of the first six nurses who obtained diplomas in midwifery, laying the foundation for the professionalization of nursing in India.

Missionary Nursing in India

- Missionary nursing in India played a pivotal role in the development and expansion of healthcare services across the country. Missionaries from various religious organizations, particularly Christian denominations, established hospitals, clinics, and nursing schools with the aim of providing medical care and promoting public health.
- Throughout the 19th and 20th centuries, missionary nurses worked tirelessly to address the healthcare needs of diverse communities, often in remote or underserved regions. They provided essential medical services, including primary care, maternal and child health services, and disease prevention initiatives.
- Missionary nursing also contributed to the professionalization of nursing in India. Many missionary organizations established nursing schools and training programs, offering formal education and certification for aspiring nurses. This not only helped to raise the standards of nursing practice but also provided opportunities

for women to enter the healthcare profession and gain economic independence.

- Furthermore, missionary nurses played a significant role in promoting health education and hygiene practices within local communities. They worked closely with community leaders and health authorities to implement initiatives aimed at improving sanitation, preventing the spread of infectious diseases, and raising awareness about preventive healthcare measures.

Nursing Education

Nursing education in India began with very brief period of training order lies and midwives were often chosen for this and were given a period of two to six months of closely supervised practical experience in general nursing than called 'Sick Nursing'. This was training in the hospital. The basic program for Combined General Nursing and Midwifery developed rapidly after 1871. The leaders of nursing in India realized that more and better qualified teachers and ward supervisors were needed if standards were to be maintained and nursing was to advance.

Hence, courses were set up in several places to give Indian nurses an opportunity to prepare themselves for responsible positions in hospitals and schools of nursing. Post certificate courses were first offered in Nursing Administration, Supervision and Teaching. These originated at the College of Nursing, New Delhi, the College of Nursing CMC Hospital, Vellore, and the Government General Hospital, Chennai. The first four-year Basic Bachelorette Degree Programs were established in 1946 at the College of Nursing in Delhi and Vellore. This program is now offered at a number of other colleges. In 1963 the School of Nursing in Thiruvananthapuram instituted the first two-year Post certificate Bachelor's Degree Program. Other colleges have begun this program since that time.

In recent years, as higher education for nurses has developed around the world, courses in India have developed so that the nurse can specialize in almost any subject and continue education through the level of the Master's degree to Doctorate degree. The first Master's Degree Course, a two-year Postgraduate Program, was begun in 1960 at the College of Nursing in Delhi.

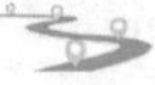

Milestones of Nursing in India

Year	*Historical Development*
1664	Military Nursing was started by East India Company in St. George Military Hospital in Chennai
1854	Government sanctioned training school for midwives
1861	Public health nursing school was started
1867	St. Stephens hospital at Delhi was first one to begin training of Indian girls as nurses
1871	First School of nursing started in Government General Hospital, Chennai with 6 months diploma midwives' program
1890-1891	Many schools under mission or government were started in various parts of India
1897	Dr BC Roy did great work in raising the standards of nursing and that of male and female nurses
1908	TNAI formed to uphold dignity and honor of nursing profession
1912	TNAI affiliated to International Nursing Council as an 8th Association in the world. In 1917 June 16th under the Registration Act No: XXI of 1860—TNAI got registered. In 1922—Student Nurses Association (SNA) formed
1918	Training schools were started for health visitors and dais at Delhi and Karachi
1926	Chennai (previously known as Madras) state formed the first registration council to provide basic standards in education and training
1946	First 4-year basic Bachelor's Degree program was established at RAK College of Nursing in Delhi and CMC, Vellore
1947	After independence, Community Development Programme and expansion of hospital service created a large demand for nurses, ANM, health visitors, midwives, nursing tutors and nursing administrators
1948	The first meeting of Indian Nursing Council (INC) was held
1950	The INC took decision to establish ANM program to meet the requirement of workers in nursing
1952	Establishment of urban field teaching center started at College of Nursing, Delhi in collaboration with existing maternal and child health (MCH) centers of Municipal Corporation, Delhi for teaching of urban community health nursing
1953	Ms Edith Buchanan, vice principal, College of Nursing (RAK), Delhi was sent to Columbia University to earn her Doctorate in Education (D. Ed.) through WHO fellowship

Year	Historical Development
1959	The first master's program in nursing was started at RAK College of Nursing, New Delhi
1963	School of Nursing in Thiruvananthapuram instituted the first 2 years post certificate Bachelor's Degree program
1963	School of Nursing in Thiruvananthapuram instituted the first 2 years post certificate Bachelor's Degree program
1985	IGNOU, established
1986	MPhil at RAK College of Nursing, New Delhi, was started
1991	The first doctoral program in nursing was established in institute of nursing sciences, MV Shetty Memorial College, Mangaluru
1992	Post basic program started under IGNOU
2002 onwards	Nursing education flourished in an unprecedented manner throughout India
2005–2006	INC started PhD program (INC consortium) with the collaboration of Rajiv Gandhi University with 25 seats

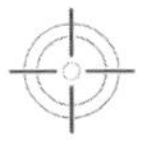

Scope of Nursing in India

The scope of nursing in India has significantly expanded over time, providing diverse career opportunities beyond traditional bedside nursing. Here are some of the career paths available for professional nurses:

- **Staff nurse:** Provides direct patient care to individuals or groups of patients in hospital or community settings. Assists in ward management and supervision under the guidance of the ward supervisor.
- **Ward sister or nursing supervisor:** Takes full charge of a ward or unit, overseeing nursing care management, assigning tasks to nursing and non-nursing personnel, and ensuring the safety and comfort of patients. Provides teaching sessions, particularly in teaching hospitals.
- **Department supervisor/assistant nursing superintendent:** Manages multiple wards or units within a specific department (e.g., surgical department, outpatient department) under the guidance of the nursing superintendent.
- **Deputy nursing superintendent:** Assists in the overall nursing administration of the hospital under the supervision of the nursing superintendent, ensuring the efficient delivery of nursing services.

- **Nursing superintendent:** Responsible for the safe and efficient management of hospital nursing services, reporting to the medical superintendent.
- **Director of nursing:** Oversees both nursing service and nursing education within a teaching hospital, ensuring high standards of patient care and professional development among nursing staff.
- **Community health nurse (CHN):** Focuses on delivering healthcare services, particularly within the scope of the Reproductive Child Health (RCH) program, in community settings. CHNs play a crucial role in promoting maternal and child health, conducting health assessments, providing preventive care, and facilitating health education programs.
- **Teaching in nursing:** The role of a nurse educator involves planning, teaching, and supervising learning experiences for students in nursing education programs. Positions in nursing education include clinical instructor, tutor, senior tutor, lecturer, associate professor, reader in nursing, and professor in nursing.
- **Industrial nurse:** Industrial nurses provide healthcare services such as first aid, illness care, and health education related to industrial hazards and accident prevention within industrial settings.
- **Military nurse:** Nurses serving in the military are commissioned officers within the Indian Army, holding ranks ranging from lieutenant to major general. They provide healthcare services to military personnel and their families.
- **Nursing service abroad:** Nurses often seek opportunities abroad due to attractive salaries and promising professional growth prospects. This trend has led to a significant increase in the number of nurses working internationally.
- **Nursing service administrative positions:** In India, nursing administrative positions range from the Deputy Director of Nursing at the state health directorate level to the Nursing Advisor to the Government of India, holding the highest administrative position at the national level.
- **Nursing leadership:** Currently, there is a shortage of strong nursing leaders in India, which hinders the advancement of the nursing profession. Effective leadership is essential for elevating the status and standards of nursing in the country. Developing competent and visionary nursing leaders is crucial for addressing

the challenges and opportunities within the healthcare system and fostering professional growth and development among nurses in India.

SUMMARY

Nursing in India has a rich history dating back to ancient times, where care for the sick and injured was provided by family members and community healers. The formalization of nursing as a profession began with the arrival of British colonial rule, which introduced Western medical practices and nursing education. The establishment of nursing schools and hospitals by missionaries and government initiatives further contributed to the growth of nursing in India.

Today, nursing in India is a diverse and dynamic field, with nurses playing crucial roles in healthcare delivery across various settings, including hospitals, clinics, community health centers, and research institutions. The profession has seen significant advancements in education, training, and specialization, with nurses taking on leadership roles and contributing to policy development and healthcare management.

Despite facing challenges such as staffing shortages, inadequate resources, and disparities in healthcare access, nurses in India continue to provide high-quality care to patients with dedication and compassion. The future of nursing in India looks promising, with ongoing efforts to improve education, training, and professional development opportunities for nurses, ensuring a strong and skilled workforce to meet the evolving healthcare needs of the country.

REVIEW QUESTIONS

Long Answer Questions

1. Discuss the scope of nursing in India.
2. Discuss the military nursing in India.

Short Answer Question

1. Enlist the milestones of nursing in India.

Multiple Choice Questions

1. In which year the bachelor's degree program is established in Delhi?
   A. 1926 B. 1936
   C. 1946 D. 1956

Ans: C. 1946

Explanation: First 4-year basic bachelor's degree program was established at RAK College of Nursing in Delhi and CMC, Vellore in 1946.

2. Where was the first school of nursing started in India?
   A. Kolkata B. Mumbai
   C. Chennai D. Delhi

Ans: C. Chennai

Explanation: In 1871, the first school of nursing was started in Government General Hospital, Madras with a six-month diploma midwives programme with four students.

3. Which of the following is the regulatory body for nursing education and practice in India?
   A. Indian Medical Association (IMA)
   B. Medical Council of India (MCI)
   C. Indian Nursing Council (INC)
   D. Nursing and Midwifery Council of India (NMCI)

Ans: C. Indian Nursing Council (INC)

Explanation: The Indian Nursing Council serves as the premier national regulatory authority overseeing nurses and nurse education within India. Established as an autonomous body under the jurisdiction of the Government of India, Ministry of Health & Family Welfare, it was instituted by the Central Government in accordance with section 3(1) of the Indian Nursing Council Act of 1947, enacted by the Indian Parliament.

Chapter 4

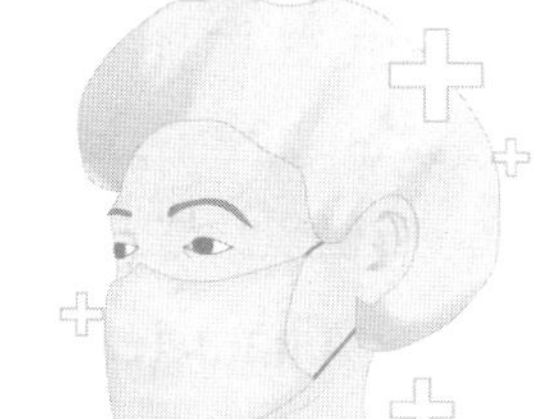

Nursing as a Profession

> *"Concentrate all your thoughts upon the work in hand. The sun's rays do not burn until brought to a focus."*
>
> ***—Alexander Graham Bell***

INTRODUCTION

Nursing is hailed as both a timeless art and a modern profession, embodying a rich historical legacy alongside contemporary advancements. It is grounded in a solid theoretical framework and encompasses a wide array of specialized skills, providing evidence-based care. Nurses undergo rigorous and continuous education, reflecting a dedication to professional growth and development. With a strong emphasis on service, nursing adheres to a comprehensive code of ethical conduct. Professional organizations serve as pillars in setting and upholding standards of practice within the profession, ensuring quality and consistency across the field.

Definitions of Profession

"Profession is a vocation require advance training and usually involving mental and manual work."

—BT Basavanthappa

"Professions are those occupations possessing a particular combination to be characteristics. Generally considered to be expertise autonomy commitment and responsibility."

—Taylor 1968

"Profession is an occupation based on specialized intellectual study and training, the purpose of which is to supply skilled service with ethical components to others, for definite fee or salary."

Characteristics of a Profession

By Abraham (1916)

- The profession involves essential intellectual operations accompanied by large undivided responsibilities.
- They are not nearly academic and theoretical but are definitely practical in their aims.
- They are self-organized with activities and duties and responsibilities which completely engage their participants and develop group consciousness.

By Willam Shepherd (1948)

- A profession must demand adequate pre-professional specialized and systematized knowledge.
- A profession must have developed a scientific technique which is the result of tested experience.
- Profession must be a type of beneficial work, the result of which is not subject to standardization in term of unit performance or time element.

By Bixler and Bixler (1959)

- A profession entrusts the educations of its practitioners to institution of higher education.
- A profession attracts individual of intellectual and personal qualities who gain and recognize their chosen occupation as life work.
- A profession constantly enlarges the body of knowledge it uses and improves to techniques of education and service by the use of scientific method.

By Kelly (1981)

- There is a special body of knowledge which is continually enlarged through research.
- There is code of ethics to guide the decisions and conduct of practitioners.
- Practitioners are relatively independently and control their own policies and activities (autonomy).

Definitions of Nursing

"Nursing means assisting the individual sick or well, in the performance those activities that will contribute to health, recovery, or a peaceful death that the individual would perform unaided, if he or she had the necessary strength, will or knowledge." ***—Virginia Henderson***

"Nursing as a special concern man's need for self-care action and the provision and management of it on a continuous basis in order to sustain life and health, recover from disease or injury and cope with their effects". ***—Dorothea Orem***

Concept of Nursing

According to EK Spalding

Nursing is a science and art dominated by ideal services, it is a science in a sense that by it utilizes the philosophy, objectives, content from medical and health sciences and is an art in the sense that it combines intelligence, observation skill and communication skill and provides services in a fine manner for the care of the individual.

PHILOSOPHY OF NURSING

The philosophy of nursing is rooted in four essential concepts: person, environment, health, and nursing. These concepts collectively shape the principles and practices of nursing, providing a comprehensive framework for understanding and addressing the needs of individuals and communities. They are interdependent, with each concept influencing and being influenced by the others, emphasizing the holistic nature of nursing care.

There are four factors involved:

1. **Nurse:** The nurse plays a primary role within the healthcare unit, demonstrating a genuine interest in their work and exuding joy while performing their duties. They adhere to systematic and orderly procedures, ensuring the correct equipment is organized before each procedure. Additionally, they diligently observe the patient's condition and promptly and accurately document relevant details.

2. **Patient:** A patient-centered approach is integral to nursing care, recognizing each patient as a holistic individual. Nurses prioritize the physical and mental comfort of patients, offering adequate explanations and providing continuous observation throughout their care to ensure high-quality service.
3. **Environmental conditions:** Creating a therapeutic environment conducive to both giving and receiving care is essential. This environment should facilitate faster recovery, characterized by cleanliness, tidiness, appropriate temperature, adequate lighting, and ventilation. Measures are taken to minimize noise and drafts, and wards or rooms are left orderly after procedures.
4. **Equipment:** Access to adequate equipment is crucial for effective patient care. Nurses ensure that all equipment used during procedures is clean and in optimal working condition. After each use, equipment undergoes thorough cleaning, sterilization, and maintenance procedures. Any malfunctioning or damaged equipment is promptly reported, and replacements are obtained as needed.

Nature and Scope of Nursing Practices

Academic study of nursing may be certificate course or degree course are detailed in **Table 4.1.**

Table 4.1: Nature and scope of nursing practice.

Nursing program	*Training duration*
Auxiliary Nurse and Midwife	2 years
General Nursing and Midwifery	3 and 1/2 years, 3 years from 2015–2016
BSc (Basic)	4 years
BSc (Post Basic)	Regular: 2 years, Distance: 3 years
MSc	2 years
MPhil	1 year (full time) and 2 years (part time)
PhD	3–5 years

Types of Nursing Professionals

Nursing personnel are among the largest number of healthcare professionals working in various fields of healthcare. They work from the lowest level of care to the highest level and in various settings, including:

- Hospital/clinical areas
- Educational settings
- Community area

Nursing Personnel in Hospital/Clinical Areas

- Nursing director
- Nursing superintendent
- Deputy nursing superintendent
- Departmental in-charge
- Head nurse
- Charge nurse
- Senior staff nurse
- Auxiliary nurse midwife
- Nursing aids

Nursing Personnel in Nursing Education

- The dean
- Principal
- Vice principal
- Reader
- Professor
- Associate professor
- Lecturer
- Assistant lecturer
- Clinical instructor

Nursing Personnel in Community Health Service

- Community health nurse
- Public health nurse
- Village health nurse
- Auxiliary nurse midwife
- Health worker—female
- Health worker—male
- Dais

Values of Professional Nursing

Professional nursing encompasses a set of core values that guide the practice and behavior of nurses. These values are essential in maintaining the integrity, effectiveness, and ethical standards of nursing care. Some of the key values of professional nursing include (**Fig. 4.1**):

- **Compassion:** Nurses demonstrate empathy, understanding, and kindness towards patients, families, and colleagues. They strive to alleviate suffering and provide comfort and support to those in need.
- **Integrity:** Nurses uphold honesty, trustworthiness, and ethical principles in all aspects of their practice. They maintain confidentiality and act with integrity in their interactions with patients and colleagues.
- **Advocacy:** Nurses serve as advocates for the health and well-being of their patients, ensuring they receive the highest quality of care and have their voices heard in decision-making processes. They advocate for patients' rights and empower them to make informed choices about their health.
- **Excellence:** Nurses strive for excellence in their practice by continually seeking to improve their knowledge, skills, and competencies. They engage in lifelong learning, evidence-based practice, and professional development to deliver the best possible care to their patients.

Values of professional nursing
• Compassion
• Advocacy
• Integrity
• Excellence
• Collaboration
• Professionalism
• Respect
• Safety

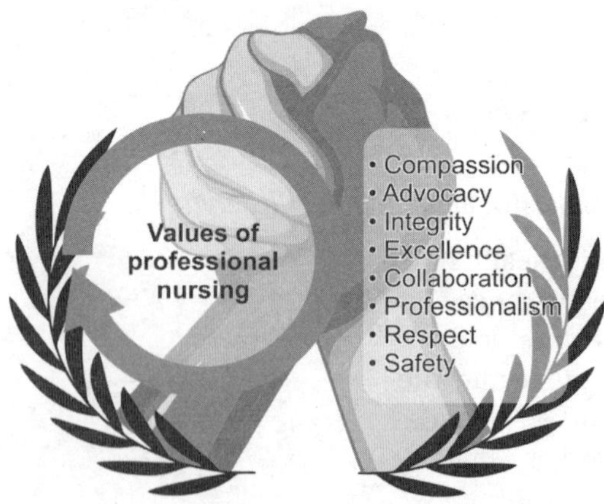

Fig. 4.1: Values of professional nursing.

- **Collaboration**: Nurses recognize the importance of teamwork and collaboration in achieving positive patient outcomes. They work effectively with interdisciplinary teams, communicating openly and respectfully with colleagues from various healthcare disciplines.
- **Professionalism:** Nurses conduct themselves with professionalism, demonstrating accountability, reliability, and ethical conduct in their interactions with patients, families, and colleagues. They adhere to professional standards and regulations governing nursing practice.
- **Respect:** Nurses show respect for the dignity, autonomy, and cultural diversity of each individual under their care. They treat patients and colleagues with dignity and courtesy, regardless of differences in background or beliefs.
- **Safety:** Nurses prioritize patient safety by implementing measures to prevent errors, minimize risks, and promote a safe healthcare environment. They follow established protocols and guidelines to ensure the well-being and security of patients and staff.

Objectives of Nursing

- To instill values of compassion, empathy, and professionalism in nursing practice, ensuring the delivery of patient-centered care with dignity and respect.
- To develop critical thinking and problem-solving skills in nurses, enabling them to assess complex healthcare situations, make informed decisions, and adapt to changing patient needs.
- To foster cultural competence and sensitivity among nurses, promoting understanding and appreciation of diverse backgrounds, beliefs, and values to provide culturally competent care.
- To promote lifelong learning and continuous professional development among nurses, encouraging them to stay updated on best practices, advancements in healthcare technology, and evidence-based research to improve patient outcomes.
- To prepare nurses to be effective communicators, both verbally and nonverbally, fostering therapeutic relationships with patients, families, and healthcare team members to facilitate optimal care delivery.

- To advocate for health equity and social justice, addressing disparities in healthcare access and outcomes, and promoting policies that support the health and well-being of all individuals and communities.
- To contribute to the advancement of nursing knowledge and research through participation in scholarly activities, including research projects, publications, and presentations, to enhance evidence-based practice and innovation in nursing care.
- To cultivate leadership skills in nurses, empowering them to take on leadership roles within healthcare organizations, professional associations, and communities to influence positive change and promote nursing excellence.
- To prioritize patient safety and quality improvement initiatives, fostering a culture of continuous improvement, risk reduction, and adherence to evidence-based standards to enhance the overall quality and safety of patient care delivery.

Basic Nursing Principles

In the curriculum of nursing schools, there is a comprehensive focus on integrating knowledge and skills across six key areas of science. This preparation equips nurses with the necessary competence to adhere to fundamental nursing principles during their practice. When executing any procedure, it is imperative to seamlessly integrate knowledge and skill to uphold the following principles:

- Safety
- Therapeutic effectiveness
- Comfort
- Uses of resources
- Good workmanship
- Individuality

Qualities of Professional Nurse

Devotion is indeed a paramount quality for anyone considering nursing as a profession, requiring meticulous care and consideration. Maintaining impassiveness is equally crucial, ensuring that nurses remain calm and composed even amidst the most challenging situations. **Figure 4.2** shows some other indispensable qualities of a nurse.

Integrity
Optimistic outlook
Loyality
Gentleness and quietness
Qualities of professional nurse
Discipline
Observation and adaptibility
Courtsey
Patience and tactful
Dignity

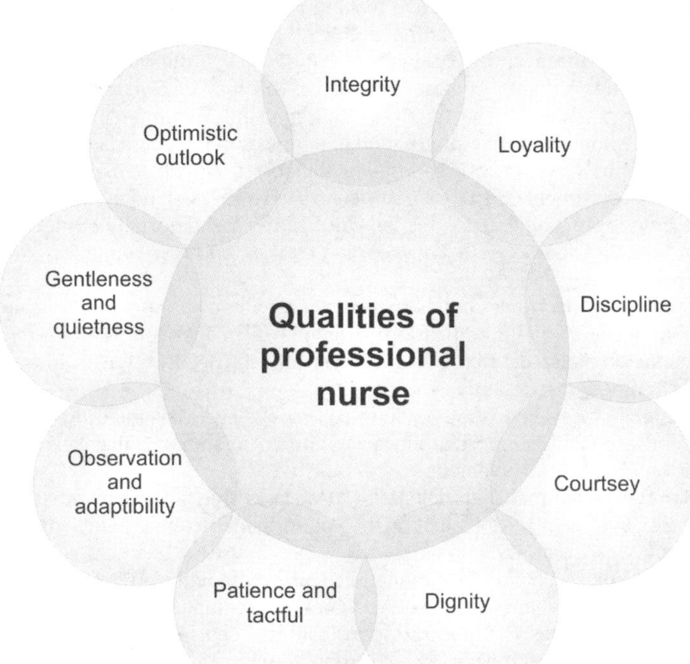

Fig. 4.2: Qualities of professional nurse.

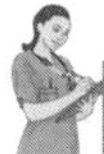

Role and Functions of a Nurse

Nurses undertake various roles simultaneously when delivering patient care, with these roles often overlapping. For instance, a nurse may act as a counselor while administering physical care and providing educational guidance (**Fig. 4.3**).

- **Caregiver:** Traditionally, the caregiver role involves assisting patients physically and psychologically while upholding their dignity. Caregiving encompasses support across physical, psychological, developmental, cultural, and spiritual dimensions.
- **Communicator:** In the role of communicator, nurses identify patient problems and effectively convey them verbally or in writing to other members of the healthcare team. Clear and accurate communication is vital for meeting the client's healthcare needs effectively.
- **Teacher:** In the role of a teacher, the nurse facilitates the client's understanding of their health condition and the necessary healthcare procedures for restoring or maintaining their well-being. This involves assessing the client's learning needs and readiness, collaboratively setting specific learning

objectives, employing effective teaching strategies, and evaluating the client's comprehension and progress.

- **Client advocate:** In the role of a client advocate, the nurse serves to safeguard the client's interests and needs. This may involve representing the client's wishes and preferences to other healthcare professionals, such as conveying the client's information preferences to the physician.
- **Counselor:** Nurses provide counseling primarily to individuals experiencing normal adjustment difficulties. Counseling focuses on assisting the individual in developing new attitudes, emotions, and behaviors by exploring alternative approaches, acknowledging choices, and fostering a sense of empowerment and control.
- **Change agent:** Nurses act as change agents when supporting clients in making behavioral modifications. They may also advocate for systemic changes in clinical care to better serve clients' health needs, as the healthcare environment is constantly evolving.
- **Leader:** Nurses demonstrate leadership at various levels, including individual client care, family support, group facilitation, collaboration with colleagues, and community involvement.
- **Manager:** Nurse managers delegate nursing tasks to ancillary staff and fellow nurses, overseeing and evaluating their performance to ensure efficient and effective care delivery.
- **Case manager:** Nurse case managers collaborate with multidisciplinary healthcare teams to assess the effectiveness of case management plans and monitor outcomes. The specific responsibilities of a nurse case manager may vary depending on the healthcare setting or unit.
- **Research consumer:** Nurses utilize research to enhance client care. This involves understanding the research process, respecting human subjects' rights, identifying researchable problems, and critically evaluating research findings to inform evidence-based practice.
- **Expanded career roles:** Nurses are increasingly assuming expanded career roles, such as nurse practitioners, clinical nurse specialists, nurse midwives, nurse educators, nurse researchers, and nurse anesthetists, reflecting the diverse opportunities available within the nursing profession.

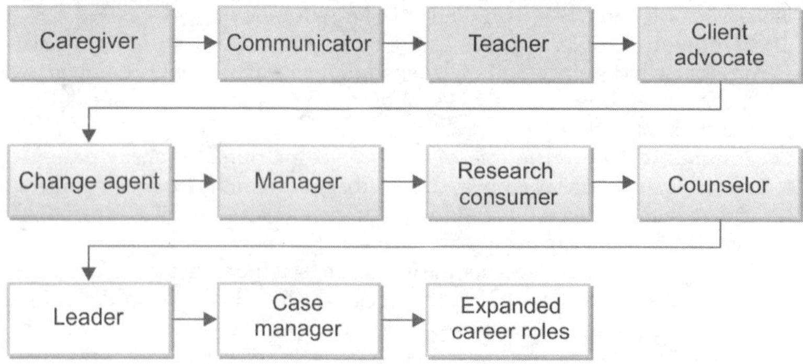

Fig. 4.3: Role and functions of a nurse.

Issues Related to Nursing Profession

- **Shortage of nurses:** Many regions worldwide are experiencing a shortage of qualified nurses, which strains healthcare systems and compromises patient care.
- **Staffing ratios:** Inadequate nurse-to-patient ratios contribute to heavy workloads, increased stress, and potential patient safety risks.
- **Workplace violence:** Nurses face a higher risk of workplace violence, including physical assaults, verbal abuse, and harassment, which can lead to physical and emotional harm.
- **Burnout and stress:** Nursing is inherently stressful, and burnout rates among nurses are alarmingly high due to long hours, emotionally taxing situations, and heavy workloads.
- **Professional development:** Continuing education opportunities are essential for nurses to maintain competence and keep up with advancements in healthcare, but access to such opportunities can be limited.
- **Scope of practice:** Legal and regulatory limitations on nursing practice can hinder nurses' ability to provide comprehensive care and fully utilize their skills and expertise.
- **Ethical dilemmas:** Nurses frequently encounter ethical dilemmas in patient care, such as issues related to autonomy, beneficence, and justice, which require careful consideration and navigation.
- **Diversity and inclusion:** There is a need for greater diversity and inclusion within the nursing workforce to better address the needs of diverse patient populations and reduce healthcare disparities.
- **Technological advancements:** While technology offers opportunities to improve patient care, nurses may face challenges related to the integration and use of technology in healthcare settings.
- **Advocacy and policy:** Nurses play a crucial role in advocating for patient rights, healthcare policy changes, and improvements to healthcare systems, but they may encounter barriers to effective advocacy and policy engagement.

SCOPE OF NURSING

The scope of nursing in India is vast and continually evolving, encompassing a wide range of opportunities and responsibilities across various healthcare settings. Some key aspects of the scope of nursing in India include:

- **Clinical practice:** Nurses play a crucial role in direct patient care across diverse healthcare settings, including hospitals, clinics, community health centers, nursing homes, and home healthcare settings. They provide comprehensive care, including assessment, diagnosis, planning, implementation, and evaluation of patient care interventions.
- **Specialty areas:** Nursing offers opportunities for specialization in various clinical areas such as critical care, pediatric nursing, maternal-child health, mental health, oncology, geriatrics, and surgical nursing. Nurses can pursue advanced training and certification to become specialists in their chosen field.
- **Education and research:** Nursing education and research are integral components of the profession. Nurses can pursue academic careers as educators, teaching future generations of nurses in academic institutions. Additionally, nurses contribute to research initiatives aimed at advancing nursing knowledge, improving patient care outcomes, and addressing healthcare challenges.
- **Advanced practice roles:** Advanced practice nurses, such as nurse practitioners, clinical nurse specialists, nurse anesthetists, and nurse midwives, have an expanded scope of practice with advanced clinical skills and specialized knowledge. They provide autonomous care, diagnose and manage health conditions, prescribe medications, and collaborate with other healthcare professionals to deliver comprehensive care.
- **Public health and community nursing:** Nurses play a vital role in public health and community-based healthcare initiatives, focusing on health promotion, disease prevention, and improving access to healthcare services. They work in collaboration with communities, government agencies, and nonprofit organizations to address public health issues and promote population health.
- **Management and leadership:** Nursing leadership roles encompass positions in nursing administration, healthcare management, and healthcare policy development. Nurse managers oversee nursing departments, coordinate patient care services, manage resources, and ensure quality and safety standards are met. Nurses

also contribute to healthcare policy development, advocating for nursing's role in shaping healthcare delivery systems.

- **Global opportunities:** With increasing globalization and demand for healthcare professionals worldwide, Indian nurses have opportunities to work internationally in countries facing shortages of healthcare workers. Many Indian nurses choose to pursue employment opportunities abroad, contributing their skills and expertise to global healthcare initiatives.

Overall, the scope of nursing in India is diverse and dynamic, offering a wide range of career opportunities for individuals passionate about healthcare and committed to making a difference in the lives of others.

SUMMARY

Nursing is a respected and essential profession that focuses on promoting health, preventing illness, and providing care to individuals of all ages and backgrounds. Nurses play a crucial role in healthcare delivery by assessing patients, developing care plans, administering treatments, and advocating for their well-being. Nursing requires a combination of clinical skills, critical thinking, compassion, and communication to effectively meet the diverse needs of patients. The profession offers a wide range of career opportunities, including specialties such as pediatrics, geriatrics, mental health, and critical care. Nurses work in various settings, including hospitals, clinics, schools, community health centers, and research institutions, collaborating with interdisciplinary teams to deliver holistic care. Nursing as a profession continues to evolve with advancements in technology, research, and healthcare policies, emphasizing the importance of evidence-based practice, lifelong learning, and professional development. Nurses are valued members of the healthcare team, making a significant impact on the well-being of individuals, families, and communities worldwide.

REVIEW QUESTIONS

Long Answer Questions

1. Define nursing. Write about the roles of a professional nurse.
2. List down the qualities of a professional nurse.

Short Answer Questions

1. Discuss the scope of nursing practice.
2. What are the characteristics of a profession?

Multiple Choice Questions

1. What distinguishes nursing as a profession from other occupations?
   A. Nursing primarily involves performing routine tasks without autonomy
   B. Nursing requires minimal education and training
   C. Nursing is guided by a code of ethics and involves specialized knowledge and skills
   D. Nursing is solely focused on physical care and does not involve emotional support for patients

Ans: C. Nursing is guided by a code of ethics and involves specialized knowledge and skills

Explanation: Nursing is considered A profession because it is characterized by the application of specialized knowledge and skills, which are guided by a professional code of ethics. This distinguishes nursing from other occupations and emphasizes its commitment to providing holistic care to individuals and communities.

2. What is the primary objective of nursing care?
   A. Providing medication administration
   B. Ensuring patient safety
   C. Facilitating patient recovery and promoting optimal health outcomes
   D. Documenting patient information

Ans: C. Facilitating patient recovery and promoting optimal health outcomes

Explanation: The primary objective of nursing care is to facilitate patient recovery and promote optimal health outcomes. This involves providing holistic care, addressing physical, emotional, social, and spiritual needs, and empowering patients to achieve their highest level of well-being.

3. Which of the following is a primary role and function of a nurse?
   A. Performing administrative tasks
   B. Conducting medical research
   C. Providing direct patient care
   D. Managing hospital finances

Ans: C. Providing direct patient care

Explanation: One of the primary roles and functions of a nurse is to provide direct patient care, which includes assessing, planning, implementing, and evaluating nursing care to meet the physical, emotional, social, and spiritual needs of patients.

Chapter 5

Development of Nursing Education in India

> *"All that we are is the result of what we have thought. The mind is everything. What we think we become."* —***Gautama Buddha***

INTRODUCTION

Nursing education in India has evolved from its early beginnings to become a structured and comprehensive discipline. Historically, nursing education in India was influenced by colonial-era practices, with the establishment of nursing schools primarily by British missionaries and colonial authorities. These early institutions focused on providing basic nursing skills to meet the healthcare needs of the time. Overall, the development of nursing education in India reflects a commitment to meeting the evolving healthcare needs of society while upholding high standards of professionalism and competence among nurses. Continued collaboration between educational institutions, regulatory bodies, healthcare providers, and policymakers will be essential in further advancing the field of nursing education in the country. A brief sketch of the developments in nursing education is given below.

EVOLUTION OF NURSING EDUCATION IN INDIA

Auxiliary Nurse Midwives

- The introduction of the Auxiliary Nurse Midwives (ANM) program in India has been a significant development in expanding healthcare services, particularly in rural areas. Initially, the 2-year ANM course was initiated in 1901 at St. Mary's Hospital Tan Taram in Punjab to address the shortage of professional nurses and provide essential healthcare services at the grassroots level.

- ANMs are trained in midwifery, basic nursing skills, and are oriented towards public health and family planning. They play a crucial role in maternal and child health (MCH) and family planning services, with responsibilities extending to areas with populations of up to 10,000. ANMs are considered the backbone of rural healthcare services in India, operating primarily from primary health centers and subcenters.
- Over the years, various committees and reports, including the Mudaliar Committee (1961), Kartar Singh Committee (1973), and Shrivastav Committee (1975), have highlighted the importance of ANMs in rural healthcare and recommended measures to enhance their effectiveness.
- One significant shift in the ANM program came with the decision to transition ANMs into multipurpose health workers (female) to broaden their scope of practice and meet the evolving healthcare needs of rural communities. This transition involved providing existing ANMs with an orientation course to equip them with additional knowledge and skills required for multipurpose roles. Additionally, the duration of the training program was reduced to 18 months from the original 2 years.
- As part of this transition, the nomenclature of ANM was changed to health worker (female) in many states, reflecting their expanded roles and responsibilities beyond traditional midwifery and nursing tasks.
- The goal of these changes was to ensure equitable access to healthcare services by deploying trained health workers (female) in rural areas, with a target of one health worker (female) for every 5,000 population by the end of the sixth Five-Year Plan.
- Overall, the evolution of the ANM program underscores India's commitment to strengthening primary healthcare services and improving health outcomes, particularly in underserved rural communities.

Lady Health Visitors

- Health visitors play a crucial role in community health by focusing on home visits and providing essential healthcare services. The establishment of the first school for health visitors, the Lady Reading Health School, in Delhi, in 1918 marked a significant milestone in recognizing the importance of community-based nursing. Subsequently, similar schools were established across the country to train health visitors.

- The training program for Lady Health Visitors (LHVs) typically lasts for 2.5 years and is based on a modified curriculum from the auxiliary nurse midwives (ANMs) course, with a stronger emphasis on maternal and child health and family planning.
- In response to evolving healthcare needs and recommendations from committees like the Kartar Singh Committee (1973) and the Shrivastav Committee (1975), the Ministry of Health, Government of India, initiated a plan of action in 1976 to adapt the roles of health visitors to the changing healthcare landscape.
- Under this plan, existing health visitors are being retrained for 16 weeks to prepare them as multipurpose workers, designated as Health Assistants (female), to better function within the country's new rural healthcare system. These Health Assistants (female) will play a supervisory role, overseeing the work of four health workers (female) within the new setup.
- For new entrants into the profession, the suggested duration of training is two years, ensuring that they are equipped with the necessary skills and knowledge to fulfill their roles effectively within the evolving healthcare system.
- Overall, the adaptation of health visitors into Health Assistants (female) reflects the government's commitment to optimizing the healthcare workforce and improving healthcare delivery, particularly in rural areas where community-based healthcare is essential for addressing the health needs of the population.

Public Health Nurses

- The Bhore Committee, in its report in 1946, advocated for the transition from partially trained workers like health visitors to more proficient public health nurses to enhance the efficiency of health services. Subsequently, in 1956, the Indian Nursing Council (INC) recommended to the States that training programs for health visitors be discontinued. Instead, they suggested incorporating all nursing content into the basic curriculum so that trained nurses could function effectively both as public health nurses in the community and as staff nurses in hospitals.
- The Mudaliar Committee in 1961 echoed similar sentiments, expressing concerns about the adequacy of the training provided to health visitors considering the responsibilities associated with their roles. They recommended replacing the existing cadre of health visitors with more qualified public health nurses.

- As a result of these recommendations, many schools of nursing integrated public health components into their basic nursing and midwifery courses. This integration aimed to equip nurses with the necessary skills and knowledge to fulfill broader public health roles while also meeting the demands of hospital-based nursing practice.
- Overall, the shift towards training nurses as public health nurses rather than health visitors reflects a commitment to improving the quality and efficiency of healthcare services, both within communities and hospital settings. By integrating public health into nursing education, nurses are better prepared to address the diverse health needs of individuals, families, and communities across the country.

General Nursing and Midwifery

- The history of nursing education in India traces back to significant milestones that have shaped the profession into what it is today. The Government of Madras took the pioneering step in 1871 by initiating the training of nurses. Subsequently, from 1874 to 1889, Christian Mission Hospitals played a pivotal role in training Indian women as nurses, making remarkable contributions despite societal challenges.
- During this period, Christian women were among the first to embrace nursing as a profession, as cultural barriers hindered Muslim girls due to the Purdah system, and Hindu girls were reluctant due to perceived social stigmas associated with nursing. However, a national movement began to emerge, spurred by the efforts of Lady Dufferin, advocating for the education of doctors, nurses, and midwives.
- The establishment of the national association in 1885 marked a significant turning point, leading to the creation of voluntary hospitals known as "Dufferin Hospitals" across the country, which also served as training schools for midwives and nurses. Initially, each hospital independently conducted training and awarded certificates, but efforts were made to standardize nursing education.
- In 1893, doctors and nursing superintendents collaborated to develop a curriculum for a three-year training course, leading to the formation of the North India United Board of Examiners

for Mission Hospitals in 1910. Similar initiatives in South India and Central Provinces led to the formation of separate boards for nursing examinations, setting the stage for standardized nursing education.

- The establishment of nursing councils in various regions, such as the Bombay Nursing Council in 1935 and the Nursing Council in Chennai in 1926, further contributed to the regulation and standardization of nursing education. By 1949, the INC was formed to ensure uniform standards across the country.
- Today, the INC continues to play a vital role in updating nursing curricula to align with evolving healthcare policies and needs, such as primary healthcare and universal health coverage. Through these ongoing efforts, nursing education in India continues to evolve to meet the diverse needs of individuals, families, and communities across the country.

Post basic Courses

- The inception of Post Basic Certificate Courses at the national level began with programs in administration and teaching, initiated in Delhi in 1943. Subsequently, in 1952, the All India Institute of Hygiene and Public Health, Kolkata, introduced the first 10-month course in public health nursing for trained nurses. Following this, several other states adopted similar programs, offering courses in public health for trained nurses.
- In addition to public health nursing, Post Basic Certificate Courses have expanded to include various other specialties. Some states now offer programs in administration, teaching, psychiatric nursing, and pediatric nursing, among others. These courses aim to provide advanced training and specialized skills to practicing nurses, enabling them to meet the diverse healthcare needs of the population.
- The introduction of Post Basic Certificate Courses reflects a commitment to enhancing the capabilities of nurses and ensuring quality healthcare delivery across different healthcare settings. By offering specialized training in key areas of nursing practice, these courses contribute to the professional development and advancement of nurses, ultimately improving patient outcomes and healthcare outcomes as a whole.

BSc Nursing

- University education for nurses was introduced in 1946, marking a significant milestone in the professionalization of nursing in India. Degree courses (BSc) were inaugurated at the College of Nursing in Vellore and New Delhi, paving the way for the establishment of more colleges of nursing offering degree programs across the country.
- The admission requirements typically include completion of pre-university or higher secondary education with a focus on science subjects. Following admission, students undergo a four-year degree course in general nursing and midwifery, equipping them with comprehensive knowledge and skills essential for nursing practice.
- In 1973, the Punjab University, in collaboration with its affiliated colleges of nursing in Chandigarh and Ludhiana, took a pioneering step by introducing a three-year BSc (Nursing) course. This program incorporated a unique clinical experience component, including a nine-month internship. During this internship period, students gain hands-on experience by working at primary health centers and immersing themselves in rural communities for eight weeks. This innovative approach to nursing education reflects a commitment to providing students with practical exposure to real-world healthcare settings, preparing them to address the diverse healthcare needs of the population.
- Overall, the introduction of university-based nursing education has played a crucial role in elevating the status of nursing as a profession and ensuring that nurses receive rigorous academic training. By integrating theory with practical experience, these programs empower nurses to deliver high-quality, evidence-based care across various healthcare settings, thereby contributing to the overall improvement of healthcare delivery in India.

MSc Nursing

- The university of Delhi introduced a course of MSc in nursing in 1960. This is a two-year course after BSc nursing. It builds upon and extend competence acquired at the graduate levels, emphasize applications of relevant theories into nursing practice, education, administration and development of results skills. Encourages accountability and commitment to lifelong learning which fosters improvement of quality care.

- The aim of the postgraduate program in nursing is to prepare graduates to assume responsibilities as nurse specialists, consultants, educators, administrators in a wide variety of professional settings.
- **Eligibility criteria:** A registered midwife of equivalent with any state nursing registration council. The minimum educational requirements shall be passing of BSc nursing/BSc Hons nursing/ Post Basic BSc nursing with minimum of 55% aggregate marks. Minimum 1 year of work experience prior or after Post Basic BSc Nursing.

PhD Nursing

- PhD programs in nursing in India began to emerge as part of the global movement towards advanced education in healthcare disciplines. While the specific date and location of the inception of PhD nursing programs in India may vary, significant developments took place in the late 20th and early 21st centuries. Notable institutions such as the All India Institute of Medical Sciences (AIIMS) in New Delhi and various universities across the country have pioneered the establishment of PhD nursing programs.
- These programs aim to cultivate nurse scholars, researchers, and educators equipped with the necessary skills and knowledge to contribute to the advancement of nursing science, evidence-based practice, and healthcare policy in India. Through rigorous research and scholarly inquiry, PhD nursing programs in India play a crucial role in shaping the future of nursing practice and education in the country.

Nurse Practitioners Programs

- Nurse practitioners can treat both physical and mental conditions through comprehensive history taking, physical exams and ordering tests for interpretation.
- Nurse practitioners can provide a diagnosis and recommendations for a wide range of acute and chronic diseases and provide appropriate treatment for patients, including prescribing medications in some states.
- Nurse practitioners can serve as a patients primary health provider, and see patients of all ages depending on their specialities. The core philosophy of the field is individualized care that focuses on

patients conditions as well as the effects of illness on the lives of the patients and their families.

- According to the International Council of nurses, A Nurse practitioners/advanced practice nurse is "a registered nurse who has acquired the knowledge base, decision making skills and clinical competencies for expanded practice beyond that of an RN, the characteristics of which would be determined by the context in which he/she is credential to practice."

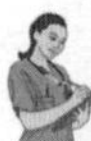

Role of Nurse Practitioner

- Medical diagnosis, treatment, evaluation and management of acute and chronic illness and disease.
- Obtaining medical histories and conducting physical examinations.
- Ordering and performing diagnostic studies (e.g., lab test, X-rays and ECGs).
- Requesting physical therapy, occupational therapy, and other rehabilitation treatments
- Prescribing drugs for acute and chronic illness
- Providing prenatal care and family planning services.
- Providing well-childcare, including screening and immunization.
- Providing primary and speciality care services, health—maintenance care for adults, including annual physicals.
- Providing care for patients in acute and critical care.
- Performing or assisting in minor surgeries and procedures (suturing, casting).
- Counseling and educating patients on heath behaviors, self-care skills and treatment options in coordination with occupational therapists and other healthcare providers.

Specialities

- Acute care nurse practitioner
- Adult nurse practitioner
- Family practice nurse practitioner
- Psychiatric nurse practitioner
- Geriatric nurse practitioner
- Pediatric nurse practitioner
- Obstetric nurse practitioner
- Neonatal nurse practitioner

- Emergency nurse practitioner
- Hepatology nurse practitioner

Practice Setting

Community clinics, health centers, urgent care centers, health maintenance organizations, home healthcare agencies, hospitals, hospital clinics, hospice care, physician offices, nursing homes, private and public schools, universities and colleges, veteran's administration facilities, retail-based clinics, bedside nursing in hospitals and walk-in-clinics.

Outline of Nursing Education in India

There are as many as eight types of training programs, which are rather confusing. There is no clear demarcation as to the levels of responsibility for each category of nursing personnel.

Demands of nurses is ever-expanding, especially in the light of newer concepts such as providing primary health care to the rural populations. The present diploma course of 3½ years duration conducted by hospital nursing schools is considered inadequate. It is increasingly realized that good nursing education has to be interdisciplinary and integrated system of education. The WHO Expert Committee on Nursing (1966) recommended that the education for nurses should be absorbed into the system of higher education of the country either in a university in through a pattern similar to that serving other professions.

Nursing of Cross Roads

The current view of nursing experts in this country is that nursing education should be brought within the mainstream of education. There is a strong opinion that, for the advancement of nursing education, schools of nursing should be separated from nursing service administration and placed under a separate department of nursing education. The recent 10+2+3 system of education recommended by the government of India has been suggested as a suitable framework into which nursing education in the country, viz, Basic nurse (+2) and Graduate nurse (+3). The entire responsibility for building up the graduate courses rest with university. Nursing education is indeed at cross roads, trying to break with some of its older traditions and altering existing stage-types.

Continuing Education

It is often said that a hospital is as good as its nursing services. Therefore, ongoing education programs are absolutely necessary for the growth of nursing and improved patient care. The International Council of Nurses and the International Labour Organization have stressed the importance of continuing education and training for nurses both at the workplace and outside, to ensure the updating and upgrading of knowledge and skills of nursing personnel and there by improve the quality of nursing care. Continuing education comprises a wide spectrum of educational activities such as staff directed individual study, in service program. Post basic courses and postgraduate academic studies are important for all levels of nursing personnel. The Raj Kumari Amrit Kaur College of Nursing, New Delhi, has in fact a separate department of continuing education for nurses.

Research in Nursing

Leaders in nursing profession are giving serious thought to promotion of research in nursing. Research is needed to acquire new knowledge and to improve both professional education and existing nursing practices. Research cannot be done in a vacuum. It requires expert knowledge in nursing, expertise in research methodology and knowledge of related sciences such as sociology, psychology, anthropology and management sciences. In other words, research in nursing like research in other fields is interdisciplinary and needs coordination with a number of other departments such as the departments of medicine, social sciences, statistics and management sciences. The Raj Kumari Amrit Kaur College of Nursing, New Delhi, has established a Department of Nursing Research in Cooperation with WHO. One of the objectives of the department is to heighten nurses awareness of research and to create an atmosphere of research consciousness among nurses at all levels in India.

Nursing Audit

If the quality of nursing has to improve there must be some sort of what is known as professional accountability. This is known as nursing audit. During the past few years, there has been an increased emphasis on nursing audit and standardization of nursing practice in the Western countries. The purpose of nursing audit is to identify the deficiencies in nursing practice and take remedial steps to improve the quality of nursing. This raises the question of nursing standards (on yard sticks against which assessment can be made). Nursing Registration Councils and National Nursing Associations are existing on certain minimum standards which each nurse is expected to maintain while providing patient care. Such standards are already existing in some countries. Leaders in nursing profession in India are seized with this problem. The nursing audit should relate to three elements in the nursing system viz, (a) content of nursing care, (b) structure of care (that is adequacy of facilities, equipment, manpower resources) and (c) outcome of nursing care, that is, end results can change in the health status of the recipients of nursing care. Nursing audit, as and when introduced, will be a historic milestone in the history of nursing in this country.

Current Trends in Nursing

- Genetics nurse
- Stem cell technology nurse
- Robots to assist, not replace
- Gps tracking
- Wireless patient monitoring
- Intelligent alarms
- Holistic nursing: Back to the future

NURSING AND MIDWIFERY COUNCIL (NMC)

Indian Nursing Council

The Indian Nursing Council was established under an Act of Parliament, known as the Indian Nursing Council Act, 1947 following a recommendation made by the Bhore Committee in 1946. The Act was subsequently amended in 1950 and 1957. The INC was constituted in 1949. Section 3(1) of the INC Act describes the constitution and composition of the council. There are 25 elected members through different registration councils and institutions, 26 ex-offices members including superintendent of nursing service and Directors of Health Services of various states, 4 nominated members of the Government of India and 3 elected members of Parliament, making a total of 55 members. The 55 members include 31 nurses, 19 doctors and 5 others. The President and Vice-Presidents are elected by the Council.

Secretary is usually the nursing advisor of the Directorate General of Health Services.

The Executive Committee consists of 7 elected members of the council. The President and Vice-President are ex-officio members. The official address of the INC is: INC, Combined Councils Building, Temple Lane, Kotla Road, New Delhi. The council meets once a year, and the executive more frequently.

The functions of the council are:

1. Prescribing minimum syllable for the training of nurses, midwives and health visitors, and regulations for the institutions conducting their courses.
2. Inspecting schools of nursing and the conduct of examinations.
3. The recognition of examining bodies.
4. The maintenance of a register of Indian nurses.

The INC has a statutory obligation to see that the minimum standards, which are prescribed are being met. In order to fulfil this function, schools of nursing are inspected, and the conduct of examinations is regulated. A report of each inspection is seen by the executive committee. The council has the power to withdraw recognition if the minimum requirements are not met. The submission of annual reports by the schools of nursing to the council is another means of exercising control to ensure that the minimum requirements laid down are met. The INC is an autonomous body and its official relationship with the state is through the state governments.

State Nursing Councils

All the states in India now have a Nursing Council. Each has its own registrar and is responsible for the registration of nurses, midwives, health visitors and auxiliary nurse midwives. Some of the state Nursing Councils are recognized as examining bodies by the INC. The state councils are legally empowered by the nurses Act to undertake responsibility to exert general supervision over the performance of the nurses within their jurisdiction. This includes checking substandard nursing service, negligence of duty and unethical behavior of registered nurses. State councils act in close cooperation with the State Governments.

Nurse Practice Act

In some countries there is a separate "Nurse Practice Act" which lays down the detailed functions which nurses of different categories in different practice areas need to perform. Such an Act will provide legal protection to nurses, and safe nursing practices for the community. The possibility of introducing such an Act in India is under active consideration.

Trained Nurses Association of India

The Trained Nurses Association is a nonsectarian, nonpolitical, professional organization whose membership in open to all registered nurses who have received a full 3-year training in general nursing and hold certificates which are recognized by the INC.

The Trained Nurses Association (TNAI) has its origin in the Association of Nursing Superintendents of India which was formed in 1905 by a small group of a nursing superintendents from different parts of the country who fall the need for and importance of the development of nursing as an honorable progression. Within 3 years, it was considered essential to enlist the cooperation of the trained nurses to advance the cause of nursing. For the reason, a second association known as the trained nurse's association of India was formed in 1908. In 1912, the TNAI was affiliated to the International Council of Nurses, in 1917 it was registered. In 1922, the two associations were amalgamated under the banner TNAI. In 1922, the student nurses association of TNAI was formed which continues to be an important wing of the TNAI.

Aims

The aims of the TNAI which are set out in its constitution are as follows:

- To uphold in every way the dignity and honor of the nursing profession.
- To promote a sense of esprit de corps among all nurses.
- To enable members to take council together, on matters affecting their professions.
- To elevate nursing education and to raise the standard of training.
- To strive to bring about a more uniform system of education, examination, certification and registration.

- To donate can subscribe to, an otherwise and any institution on organization in, or outside, India connected with nursing.
- To promote and provide for welfare of, and to give relief by grants of money on other aid, on otherwise as the association may thing fit.

Achievements

Some of the important achievements of the TNAI are: (1) raising the standard of training, of both general and midwifery, (2) the establishment of nurse registration councils in many states, (3) the establishment of the college of nursing in Delhi, (4) formation of the Health Visitor's, League, the Midwives Association and the Student Nurses Association. A detailed account of the TNAI will be found in the booklet "TNAI handbook, the TNAI in the only professional association of nurses devoted to work for the welfare of nurses throughout the country on a national level."

International Council of Nurses

The International Council of Nurses (ICN) was founded in 1899 by Mrs Bedford Fenwick, an Englishwoman. The ICN is the oldest international association of professional women. Membership is open to all self-governing national nurses associations. The INC was affiliated to the ICN in 1912. The headquarters of the ICN are located in Geneva, Switzerland. Currently, the ICN is a federation of 95 National Nurse Association representing over a million nurses throughout the world. Nurses of national association are automatically members of the ICN. Under the auspices of the ICN, nurses from national association may attend international conferences visit other countries for study, employment. On observation the rough the ICN exchange of privileges program; obtain advice and assistance through the ICN headquarters and may draw on the resources of the ICN information center. The ICN is in official relationship with the WHO, UNICEF, ILO and other international bodies. The ICN publishers a quarterly journal, the International Nursing Review. An international conference of ICN is held every four years. May 12 is usually celebrated around the world as International Nurses Day, as on this day Florence Nightingale was born founder of modern nursing. But the national association are free to choose another date of special significance to the nursing profession within their own country.

SUMMARY

Nursing education in India has undergone significant development over the years, evolving from informal training to formalized programs that meet international standards. The establishment of nursing schools and colleges, both by government and private institutions, has played a crucial role in shaping the education and training of nurses in the country. The introduction of standardized curricula, accreditation processes, and regulatory bodies such as the INC has helped ensure quality and consistency in nursing education. Additionally, advancements in technology and teaching methodologies have enhanced the learning experience for nursing students, providing them with practical skills and knowledge to meet the demands of modern healthcare settings. Specialized programs in areas such as critical care, oncology, and community health have also been introduced to cater to the diverse needs of patients and healthcare systems. Continuous efforts are being made to improve the infrastructure, faculty training, and research opportunities in nursing education, aiming to produce competent and compassionate nurses who can contribute effectively to the healthcare sector in India and beyond.

REVIEW QUESTIONS

Long Answer Question

1. Write a succinct growth of nursing education in India.

Short Answer Question

1. Write a short note on research in nursing.

Multiple Choice Questions

1. What is the primary purpose of a nursing audit?
   A. To increase healthcare costs
   B. To evaluate the quality of nursing care
   C. To reduce patient satisfaction
   D. To limit access to healthcare services

Ans. B. To evaluate the quality of nursing care

Explanation: The primary purpose of a nursing audit is to assess and evaluate the quality of nursing care provided to patients, identify areas for improvement, and ensure adherence to established standards and protocols.

2. Which of the following is a key component of a nursing audit process?
   A. Ignoring feedback from healthcare providers
   B. Focusing solely on individual performance
   C. Involving interdisciplinary collaboration
   D. Avoiding data collection and analysis

Ans. C. Involving interdisciplinary collaboration

Explanation: A key component of a nursing audit process is to involve interdisciplinary collaboration, including nurses, healthcare providers, administrators, and other stakeholders, to gather diverse perspectives and insights for a comprehensive evaluation.

Chapter 6

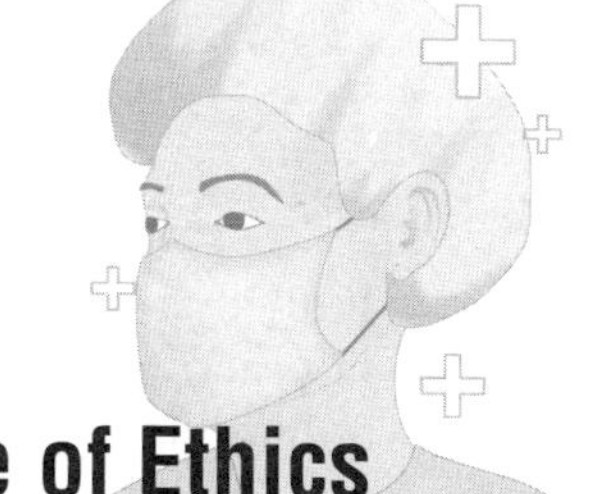

Code of Ethics

> *"If four things are followed-having a great aim, acquiring knowledge, hard work, and perseverance-then anything can be achieved."*
>
> ***—APJ Abdul Kalam***

ETHICAL ASPECTS OF NURSING

Ethics is the systematic examination of the appropriate conduct and actions concerning oneself, other individuals, and the environment. Its significance within nursing cannot be overstated. Nursing has a longstanding tradition of embracing ethical codes, moral principles, and active engagement with ethical dilemmas. Central to nursing is the provision of care and comfort to the sick while safeguarding their well-being, actions that inherently shape societal norms and values.

Nursing ethics establish the benchmarks for professional conduct, serving as the compass for navigating moral complexities. They delineate the responsibilities and commitments of nurses to their patients, colleagues, the broader healthcare community, and society at large. In essence, nursing ethics serve as a guiding framework for upholding principles of right and wrong conduct within the profession.

Furthermore, nursing ethics transcends rote adherence to rules; it nurtures deep reflection on morality, ethical deliberation, and the resolution of moral dilemmas. This involves delving into interdisciplinary realms, including philosophy and theology, to enhance nurses' abilities in moral discernment and ethical decision-making

CODE OF ETHICS

Professional codes of ethics serve as a cornerstone for guiding behavior and upholding standards within any field. They not only regulate individual conduct but also underscore the collective responsibility of practitioners towards society. In the context of nursing in India, adherence to the International Council of Nurses Code for Nurses (1993) signifies a commitment to the following principles:

- Nurses are entrusted with the fundamental duty of promoting health, preventing illness, restoring health, and alleviating suffering. These responsibilities form the bedrock of nursing practice, guiding actions aimed at enhancing the well-being of individuals and communities.
- The essence of nursing lies in its universal relevance, transcending boundaries of nationality, race, ethnicity, color, age, and socioeconomic status. Nurses are bound by a steadfast respect for human life, dignity, and rights, irrespective of cultural or societal differences.

By adhering to these principles, nurses in India uphold the integrity of their profession, fostering trust and accountability while ensuring the delivery of compassionate and ethical care to all individuals in need **(Fig. 6.1)**.

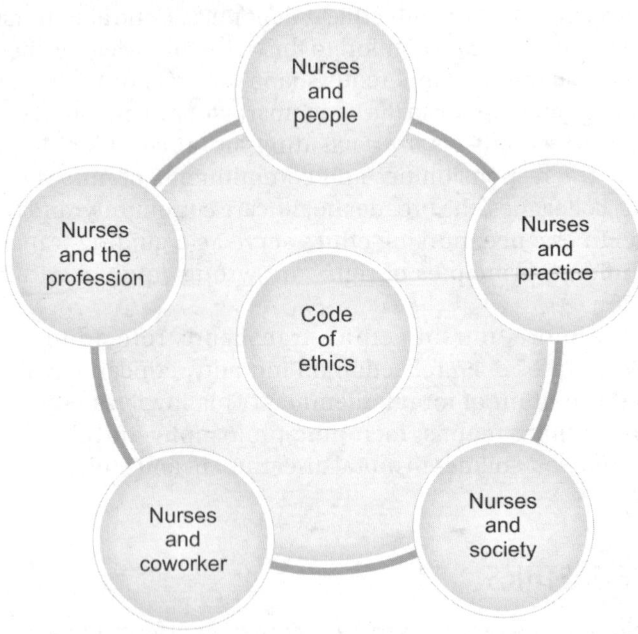

Fig. 6.1: Code of ethics.

Nurses and People

- The foremost obligation of nurses is to the individuals under their care, ensuring their well-being and addressing their healthcare needs.
- Nurses foster an environment that respects and honors the personal values, cultural customs, and spiritual beliefs of each individual.
- Nurses handle personal information with discretion, maintaining confidentiality and using judgment in sharing relevant information.

Nurses and Practice

- Nurses bear personal responsibility for their practice, continually advancing their knowledge and skills through ongoing learning.
- Upholding the highest standards of nursing care in every situation, nurses exercise judgment regarding their own competencies when accepting or delegating tasks.
- Nurses uphold a professional demeanor that reflects positively on the nursing profession at all times.

Nurses and Society

Nurses share in the collective responsibility, alongside other citizens, to advocate for and support initiatives aimed at meeting the health and social needs of the public.

Nurses and Coworker

- Nurses foster collaborative relationships not only with colleagues in nursing but also with professionals from other disciplines.
- When necessary, nurses take appropriate steps to protect individuals under their care from harm, whether it originates from coworkers or any other source.

Nurses and Profession

- Nurses play a crucial role in shaping and implementing standards of practice and education within the nursing profession.
- Actively engaging in the development and dissemination of professional knowledge, nurses contribute to the ongoing enhancement of the nursing field.

❖ Through participation in professional organizations, nurses work towards establishing fair and just working conditions, both socially and economically.

Ethical Principles

Ethical principles **(Fig. 6.2)** actually control professionalism nursing practice much more than to ethical theories. Principles encompass basic promises from which rules are developed. Principles are the moral norms that nursing, as a profession, both demands and strives to implement to every day clinical practice.

Ethical principle that the nurse should consider when making decisions are as follows:

❖ **Respect for persons:** It directs individuals to treat themselves and others with a respect inherent to man's humanness. This respect to persons needs to be simplified as it affects nursing practice.

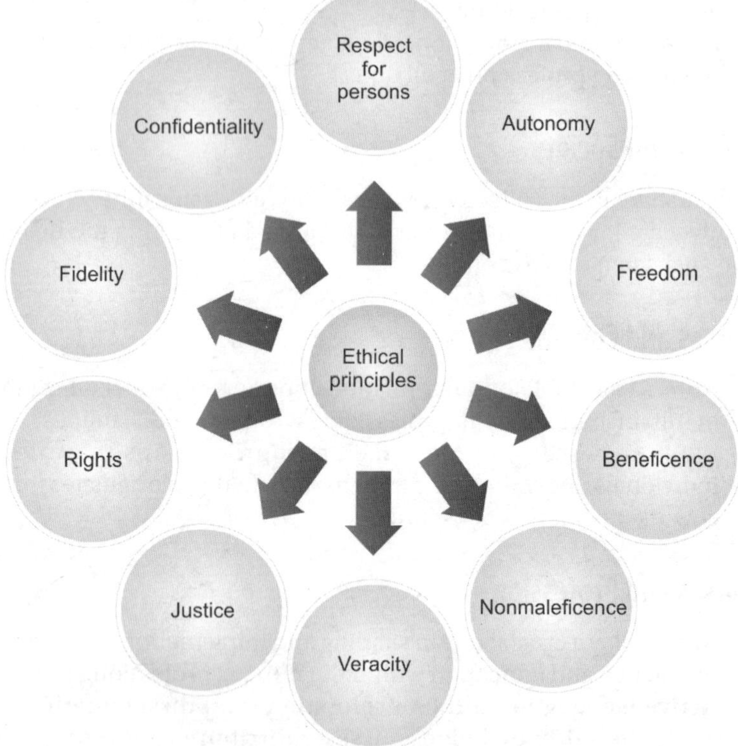

Fig. 6.2: Ethical principles.

- **Autonomy:** This principle emphasizes individuals' freedom of choice and their willingness to take responsibility for their decisions. Supported by the legal concept of self-determination, autonomy is exemplified through practices such as informed consent, where healthcare professionals must ensure patients understand their treatment options and research participation before proceeding.
- **Freedom:** The principle of individual freedom demands that patient to exempt from control by others to select and pursue personal health goals. This principle should be observed when planning patient care, by nurse manager when leading subordinates.
- **Beneficence:** Guided by the principle of beneficence, healthcare professionals are compelled to act in ways that promote the well-being of individuals. This involves carefully balancing potential harms with benefits when making decisions or taking actions.
- **Nonmaleficence:** Central to the principle of nonmaleficence is the obligation to refrain from causing harm. Nurses must interpret harm broadly, encompassing not only physical injury but also emotional and social repercussions. Despite challenges, nurses strive to minimize discomfort and pain while delivering care and performing procedures.
- **Veracity:** Veracity underscores the ethical obligation to truthfulness, requiring healthcare providers to provide patients with accurate and reality-based information about their health status. Truth-telling fosters trust between patients and caregivers, laying the foundation for hope and the expectation of benefits from nursing services.
- **Justice:** Justice revolves around the fair and equitable treatment of individuals. In healthcare, nurses are tasked with distributing limited resources in a manner that ensures equal access to care. However, complexities arise when individuals have differing needs or when resources are insufficient to provide everyone with an equal share.
- **Rights:** Rights is an entitlement to behave in a certain way under circumstances, such as nurses' entitlement to freely express personal beliefs and preferences by voting in a political election. Right is the prerogative to define another's behavior in selected situations. A right is also a claim to a specific good, service.
- **Fidelity:** Fidelity entails honoring commitments and fulfilling obligations. Nurses demonstrate fidelity by maintaining

consistency and reliability in their caregiving practices. Nurse managers also adhere to this principle by upholding promises made to employees regarding benefits, scheduling, or career advancement.

- **Confidentiality:** The principle of confidentiality underscores the duty to safeguard privileged information. Nurses respect patients' privacy rights and use personal data solely to enhance the quality of care provided. Confidentiality is essential for building trust and maintaining the therapeutic relationship between patients and healthcare providers.

By adhering to these ethical principles, nurses uphold the dignity, autonomy, and well-being of individuals under their care, fostering an environment of trust, respect, and compassion within the healthcare setting.

Ethical Issues

Nurses frequently encounter situations where they are tasked with balancing the needs and expectations of patients, physicians, and organizations, each of which may present conflicting demands, desires, and objectives.

In nursing literature, various terms are used to describe moral issues faced by nurses:

- **Moral uncertainty:** Occurs when an individual is uncertain about which moral principles or values should guide their actions, sometimes even struggling to identify the moral problem itself. This can also be referred to as moral conflict, arising when the duties and obligations of healthcare providers are unclear.
- **Moral distress:** Arises when an individual knows the right course of action but faces organizational constraints that hinder them from taking that action.
- **Moral outrage:** Occurs when an individual witnesses an immoral act by another but feels powerless to intervene and prevent it.
- **Moral/ethical dilemma**: Represents the most challenging ethical issue, involving the choice between two or more undesirable alternatives, with the aim of selecting the least damaging option.

Given that ethical dilemmas are prevalent and particularly challenging for nurse practitioners, it is essential to focus on addressing these issues.

Healthcare delivery practices pose dilemmas that vary based on how different stakeholders, including patients, healthcare agencies, legal systems, and nurses themselves, perceive the issues and potential courses of action. Nurses across all specialties encounter ethical dilemmas such as:

- Balancing the need for rational patient care with the imperative to conserve scarce resources.
- Making treatment and care decisions for terminally ill patients.
- Obtaining informed consent from patients for care and treatment.
- Responding to patient requests for assisted suicide.
- Striking a balance between patient confidentiality and privacy rights and society's need for protection from unreasonable risks.
- Safeguarding the autonomy rights of children and incompetent adults regarding research participation.
- Upholding justice by ensuring patients' rights to participate in randomized trials of experimental treatments.

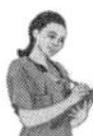

Roles and Functions of Nurse in Ethical Issues

The leadership role and management functions of an administrator in ethical issues encompass the following:

- **Self-awareness:** Administrators must possess self-awareness regarding their own values and fundamental beliefs concerning human rights, duties, and objectives.
- **Acceptance of ambiguity:** Recognizing that ethical decision-making often involves ambiguity and uncertainty, administrators are prepared to navigate such complexities.
- **Acknowledgment of negative outcomes:** Despite employing high-quality problem-solving and decision-making processes, administrators acknowledge that ethical decisions may sometimes lead to unfavorable outcomes.
- **Demonstrating risk-taking:** Administrators demonstrate willingness to take risks in ethical decision-making processes when necessary.
- **Role modeling ethical behavior:** Administrators serve as role models by consistently making ethical decisions that align with established codes of ethics and personal introspective values.
- **Advocacy:** Actively advocating for the welfare and rights of clients, employees, and fellow professionals is a key responsibility of administrators.
- **Clear communication:** Administrators clearly communicate expected standards of ethical behavior to all stakeholders.
- **Systematic problem-solving:** When faced with management issues with ethical implications, administrators utilize systematic approaches to problem-solving and decision-making.

- **Identifying outcomes:** Administrators identify outcomes in ethical decision-making that should be prioritized or avoided.
- **Framework application:** Utilizing established ethical frameworks, administrators clarify their values and beliefs to guide decision-making processes.
- **Ethical reasoning:** Applying principles of ethical reasoning, administrators define which beliefs or values form the basis of their decision-making.
- **Legal awareness:** Administrators are aware of legal precedents that may influence ethical decision-making and accept accountability for potential liabilities if decisions conflict with legal standards.
- **Recognition and rewards:** Administrators recognize and reward ethical conduct among subordinates to foster a culture of integrity.
- **Addressing unethical conduct:** Administrators take appropriate action when subordinates engage in unethical behavior, ensuring accountability and maintaining ethical standards within the organization.

SUMMARY

The code of ethics is a set of principles and guidelines that govern the behavior and conduct of individuals within a particular profession or organization. It outlines the moral obligations, values, and standards that members are expected to uphold in their interactions with clients, colleagues, and the public. The code of ethics serves as a framework for promoting integrity, professionalism, and accountability in decision-making and actions. It helps establish trust, respect, and fairness in relationships, while also protecting the rights and well-being of all parties involved. Adherence to the code of ethics is essential for maintaining the reputation and credibility of the profession or organization, as well as ensuring the highest standards of quality and ethical practice. Violations of the code of ethics may result in disciplinary actions or consequences, highlighting the importance of ethical behavior in upholding the values and mission of the profession or organization.

REVIEW QUESTIONS

Long Answer Questions

1. Write in detail about ethical principles that the nurse should consider while making decisions.
2. Explain the code of ethics in nursing.

Short Answer Questions

1. Explain the roles and functions of nurses in ethical issues.
2. Explain nurse and profession in code of ethics.

Multiple Choice Questions

1. What is the purpose of a code of ethics in nursing?
   A. To dictate strict rules and regulations for nurses
   B. To ensure nurses receive proper training and education
   C. To guide ethical decision-making and behavior among nurses
   D. To establish hierarchy within the nursing profession

Ans: C. To guide ethical decision-making and behavior among nurses.

Explanation: A code of ethics in nursing serves to provide guidelines and principles to help nurses navigate ethical dilemmas and make decisions that are in the best interest of patients and the profession.

2. Which of the following best describes the function of a code of ethics in nursing?
   A. Dictating specific protocols for patient care
   B. Providing legal regulations for nursing practice
   C. Guiding professional conduct and decision-making
   D. Establishing standards for nursing education

Ans: C. Guiding professional conduct and decision-making.

Explanation: A code of ethics in nursing serves as a framework for guiding the professional conduct and decision-making of nurses. It outlines core values, principles, and standards of behavior that nurses should uphold in their practice.

3. Which of the following is typically included in a code of ethics for nursing?
   A. Billing procedures
   B. Clinical skills training
   C. Professional values and standards of conduct
   D. Facility maintenance protocols

Ans: C. Professional values and standards of conduct

Explanation: A code of ethics for nursing typically includes professional values such as integrity, compassion, and respect, as well as standards of conduct that guide nurses in their interactions with patients, colleagues, and the community.

Chapter 7

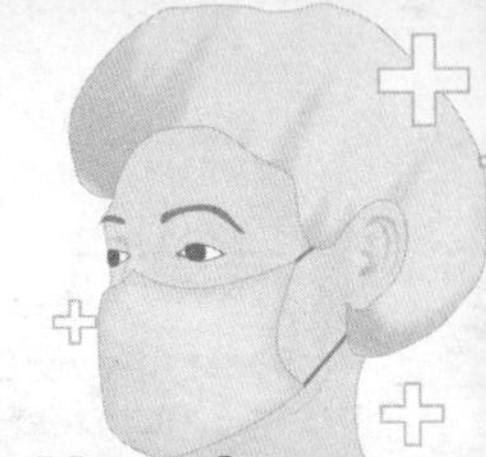

Trends in Nursing

> *"Education is the most powerful weapon which you can use to change the world."*
> —***Nelson Mandela***

INTRODUCTION

The nursing profession is undergoing continuous evolution in response to a multitude of factors, including societal needs, changing definitions of nursing, educational requirements, and expanded practice roles. Today's nurse is vastly different from those of previous decades, reflecting the ongoing development of the profession. Emerging trends and challenges are shaping the landscape of nursing, closely intertwined with broader healthcare trends. While some trends may lead to lasting changes, others may be short-lived. The current nursing shortage is a significant concern, with an anticipated national deficit of nurses posing a critical threat to the healthcare workforce. This shortage coincides with an aging population and an increase in chronic illnesses, highlighting the growing demand for skilled nursing care. Efforts such as the Reinvestment Act of 2002 aim to address the nursing shortage, expand career opportunities for nurses, and enhance governance within healthcare facilities. Adapting to these trends and challenges is essential for the nursing profession to continue delivering high-quality healthcare services.

NURSING TRENDS

A trend in nursing refers to a current change or development within the nursing field that impacts the profession. It signifies a shift or movement in a specific direction, reflecting the general directions and prevailing opinions or movements within the nursing community. Trends in nursing encompass the evolving landscape of nursing events and practices, as well as the changing attitudes and tendencies within the profession. These trends highlight the ongoing transformations and innovations taking place in various areas of nursing, including nursing services, administration, and nursing education.

Trends in Nursing Practices

Trends in nursing practices encompass a variety of dimensions that are closely linked to nurses, their roles, nursing education, and nursing services.

- **Type of nursing:** Nursing services are provided in a range of settings, including missionary, military, and civilian hospitals. Nurses care for patients in both public and private healthcare facilities, as well as engage in community-based nursing, such as in missionary, military, and railway hospital-based settings.
- **Nursing agency:** Historically, nursing care was primarily delivered by Western nurses and Christian Anglo-Indian nurses. However, over time, Indian nurses from diverse backgrounds, regardless of caste, creed, religion, or gender, have been trained to provide care to patients.
- **Focus on nursing care:** While the traditional focus of nursing care was primarily on primary nursing care, there has been a gradual shift towards emphasizing quality care and specialty care in contemporary nursing practices.
- **Nature of care:** Historically, traditional care was the primary focus, but today there is a shift towards evidence-based practice. This trend is likely to continue, with an ongoing emphasis on competency and evidence-based nursing care in the future.
- **Type of nursing care:** Currently, there is a focus on specialized nursing care, such as caring for patients with cardiovascular and respiratory conditions, in contrast to the past emphasis on general/basic nursing. Looking ahead, nurses are expected to receive training for super/subspecialty care to meet evolving healthcare needs.
- **Mode of nursing care delivery:** In the past, nursing care was predominantly delivered in person; however, there has been a transition towards distance care through teleconsultation. Moving forward, nurses are anticipated to provide care to patients using telenursing and teleconsultation methods, reflecting the evolving landscape of healthcare delivery.
- **Role of nurses:** The roles of nurses have evolved beyond traditional boundaries set by nursing practice legislation. Nurses now work

in various settings including hospitals, communities, schools, occupational environments, disaster response, home care, and more, taking on diverse nursing roles. They serve as clinical nurse specialists, primary care nurses, and nurse practitioners specializing in areas like midwifery and critical care. Nurses are expected to see further expansion in their roles, enabling them to assess patient health, provide support to patients and families across all levels of care, develop innovative evidence-based care models, deliver cost-effective quality care, and collaborate effectively within interprofessional healthcare teams to enhance the efficiency of the health system.

- **Role of nurse practitioners:** Historically, nurses held dependent roles, but the trend towards preparing nurses as independent nurse practitioners is continuing.
- **Advancement in information technology:** The present era has seen significant advancements in technology that were previously lacking. This has led to changes in nursing education curricula and practice areas. Hospitals now utilize computer-based information technology such as Hospital Information System Computerized Record Systems. Documentation is increasingly done directly on computers, often at the patient's bedside. Wireless handheld computers enable healthcare professionals to access information conveniently, even remotely. Personal digital assistants (PDAs) and electronic organizers assist nurses in managing information and time effectively. The adoption of computerized patient records, known as CPR, CMR, or OLPR, is becoming more prevalent. Nurses are required to possess comprehensive knowledge to effectively navigate and utilize advanced information and technology in their practice.
- **Interprofessional collaboration:** There is a growing emphasis on interprofessional collaboration in the nursing profession compared to the past. This trend is likely to continue and further enhance collaboration among healthcare professionals from different disciplines, leading to improved patient outcomes and holistic care.
- **Nurse administrators' leadership behavior:** Nurse administrators have shifted from autocratic leadership styles to more democratic and participatory approaches. They are now expected to exhibit transformational and transactional leadership behaviors, focusing on motivating, guiding, and supervising nurses at various levels to create a positive work environment and enhance patient care.

- **Duty pattern:** Nurses used to work in split shift duties or 8-hour shifts until the 1980s. The shift towards a straight duty shift pattern has been more convenient for nurses. This trend may continue based on hospital requirements, nursing workforce availability, and resource allocation.
- **Assignment of nurses:** In the past, nurses primarily had functional assignments. However, in the present scenario, nurses have both functional and patient assignments. In the future, there may be a shift towards assigning patients to holistic or individualized care, reflecting a more patient-centered approach to nursing care.
- **Marital status criteria:** Historically, nurses were often not allowed to marry during their training period, leading to many remaining unmarried. However, the trend shifted in the 1980s, with more married nurses opting to continue in the profession. This trend is expected to persist, allowing for a more diverse nursing workforce.
- **Uniform attire:** The traditional Western-style uniform attire for nurses, typically white with a cap, has evolved in the public sector to reflect Indian cultural norms and come in a variety of shades based on designation. There is no uniformity in uniform colors across the country, showcasing diversity and cultural sensitivity in nursing attire.
- **Nurses' preparation:** Nursing education has transitioned from on-the-job learning to formal education programs since the mid-19th century. Today, nurses receive sophisticated and specialized training through school and university-level competency-based programs like GNM and BSc nursing. There is also an emphasis on preparing nurses at master's and doctorate levels to provide specialized, evidence-based care, ensuring high-quality nursing practice and continuous professional development.
- **Number of nursing institutions:** In the past, there were limited schools/colleges offering nursing training programs. However, currently, there has been a significant increase in the number of nursing institutions, and in the future, more nursing institutions will be established to meet the growing demand for healthcare professionals.
- **Type of nursing programs:** Previously, nursing education mainly consisted of hospital-controlled diploma programs. Today, there is a wide range of nursing programs available, including Certificate, diploma, BSc, MSc, and PhD programs approved by the Indian Nursing Council (INC). Additionally, there are residency and postgraduate specialty programs. In the future, there will be a

greater emphasis on competency-based education and hybrid or e-Learning modes of learning, with a focus on simulation for teaching clinical care.

- **Mode of education:** In the past, nursing education was primarily hospital-oriented and controlled. Currently, nursing education has shifted towards institute-oriented approaches, including face-to-face and distance learning, with a minimum online component. Moving forward, there will be a greater emphasis on hybrid or e-Learning education, with a focus on simulation to enhance clinical care teaching.
- **Global health:** Historically, there was limited focus on global health in nursing education. However, there is now a growing emphasis on global health initiatives. In the future, nursing education will place even greater importance on addressing various global health issues, preparing nurses to contribute effectively to global healthcare challenges.
- **Evidence-based practice:** Although nurses have conducted and published research since 1950, only recently has the importance of nursing care been recognized. By identifying and analyzing the best available scientific evidence, nurses are steadily developing further guidelines for clinical practice that are useful nationally and internationally.
- **Scientific basis:** In the past nursing largely was either intuitive or relied on experience or observation rather than on research. Through trial and error, the individual nurses discovered with measures would assist the client and many nurses became highly skilled in providing care through experience.
- **Expansion of employment opportunities:** Nursing practice trends include a growing variety of employment setting in which you have greater independence, autonomy, and respect as a member of healthcare team. Nursing roles continue to expand and develop, broadening the focus on complementary and alternative medicine and look for a position in setting using alternative therapies. It is to remember that the opportunities are limitless for caring, compassionate, and competent nursing care; there is an area of nursing for every interest.
- **Innovations in teaching and learning/emphasis on high-tech high-touch approach:** Obtaining your nursing education online is one of the latest trends in nursing. Before, students really go to school to study nursing subjects with teachers explaining things

to them. Nowadays, Nursing students can gain their diploma by studying online, their professors demonstrate things they need to learn online, and they also get exams using the net.

It's great to see the positive changes happening in the nursing profession, such as the shift towards interprofessional collaboration and more participatory leadership among nurse administrators. The evolution of duty patterns and assignment methods also reflects a more holistic approach to patient care. The changing criteria around marital status and uniform attire show a shift towards inclusivity and cultural sensitivity. The emphasis on formal education and specialized training for nurses at all levels is crucial for providing high-quality, evidence-based care. These trends are likely to continue shaping the future of nursing in a positive direction.

Trends in Nursing Education

Nursing education is a professional education which is consciously and systematically planned and implemented through instruction and discipline and aims the harmonious development of the physical, intellectual, social, emotional, spiritual and aesthetic power or abilities of the student in order to render professional nursing care to people of all ages in all phases of health and illness, in a variety of setting in the best or highest possible manner. **Figure 7.1** depicts the different trends in nursing education.

Factors Affecting Trends in Nursing

- **Advancements in healthcare technology**: The rapid evolution of medical technology and equipment has a significant impact on the practice of nursing, requiring nurses to continually update their skills and knowledge to effectively utilize these tools in patient care.
- **Changing demographics:** Shifting demographics, such as an aging population and increasing prevalence of chronic diseases, influence the demand for nursing services and the types of care needed.
- **Healthcare policy and legislation:** Changes in healthcare policies and regulations can affect the delivery of nursing care, staffing ratios, reimbursement models, and scope of practice for nurses.

Emergence of new specialists
Educational quality assurance
Emphasis in high-tech-high touch approach
Innovations in teaching and learning
Curriculum changes
Preparation of global nurses
Transnational acceptance
Ensuring a promising career
Increased opportunities for higher studies
Diminishing government role

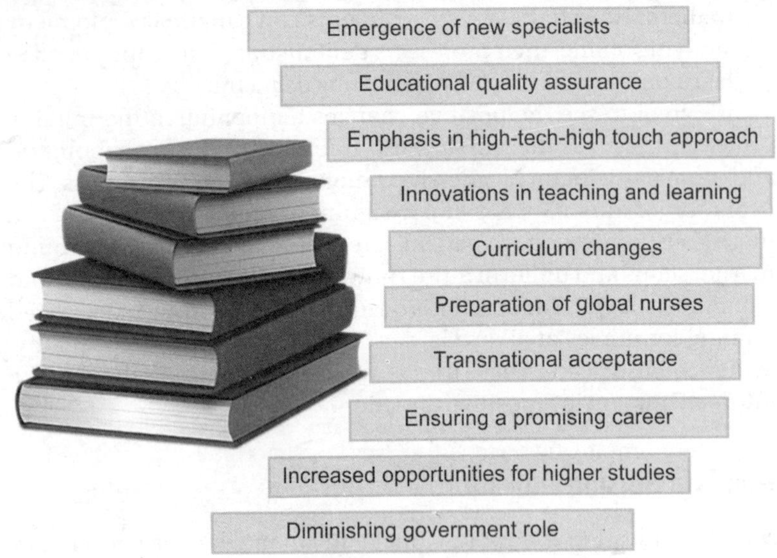

Fig. 7.1: Trends in nursing education.

- **Nursing shortages:** Shortages of qualified nurses in many regions can impact the quality of patient care, workload for existing nurses, and the need for innovative solutions to address staffing challenges.
- **Global health challenges:** Emerging infectious diseases, pandemics, and other global health issues require nurses to adapt to new care protocols, infection control measures, and public health initiatives.
- **Patient-centered care:** The emphasis on patient-centered care and shared decision-making requires nurses to enhance their communication skills, cultural competence, and ability to engage patients in their care.
- **Interprofessional collaboration:** Collaborative practice models involving nurses working with other healthcare professionals require nurses to develop teamwork skills, leadership abilities, and a holistic approach to patient care.
- **Professional development opportunities:** Access to continuing education, career advancement programs, and opportunities for specialization influence the professional growth and job satisfaction of nurses, impacting overall trends in the nursing profession.

Issues in Nursing

Nursing, as a vital component of the healthcare system, faces a myriad of challenges and issues in today's complex healthcare landscape. One of the primary issues in nursing is the ongoing shortage of qualified nurses, leading to increased workloads, burnout, and compromised patient care. Additionally, the aging population and rising prevalence of chronic diseases have placed greater demands on nurses, requiring them to provide more complex and specialized care. Another significant issue is the lack of resources and support for nurses, including inadequate staffing levels, limited access to training and professional development opportunities, and insufficient recognition of their contributions. Furthermore, issues such as workplace violence, ethical dilemmas, and the impact of technology on nursing practice add to the complexities faced by nurses in delivering high-quality care. Addressing these issues requires collaborative efforts from healthcare organizations, policymakers, and the nursing community to ensure a sustainable and supportive environment for nurses to thrive and continue providing safe and effective care to patients. Some issues are depicted in **Figure 7.2**.

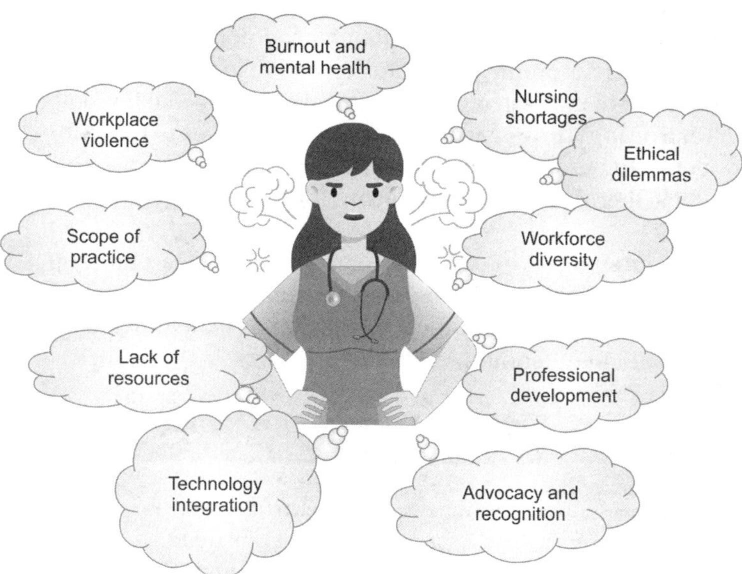

Fig. 7.2: Issues in nursing.

- **Nursing shortages:** Persistent shortages of qualified nurses in many regions lead to increased workloads, burnout, and compromised patient care quality.
- **Workforce diversity:** Lack of diversity in the nursing workforce can hinder culturally competent care delivery and limit representation of underrepresented groups in the profession.
- **Workplace violence:** Nurses often face verbal, physical, and emotional abuse from patients, families, or colleagues, leading to stress, trauma, and safety concerns.
- **Burnout and mental health:** High levels of stress, long hours, and emotional demands contribute to burnout, compassion fatigue, and mental health issues among nurses.
- **Lack of resources:** Inadequate staffing, equipment, and support systems in healthcare settings can impede nurses' ability to provide optimal care and contribute to job dissatisfaction.
- **Scope of practice:** Restrictions on nurses' scope of practice, varying by state or country, can limit their ability to practice to the full extent of their education and training.
- **Professional development:** Limited access to continuing education, career advancement opportunities, and mentorship programs can hinder nurses' professional growth and job satisfaction.
- **Ethical dilemmas:** Nurses often face ethical challenges related to patient autonomy, end-of-life care, resource allocation, and conflicts of interest, requiring ethical decision-making skills.
- **Technology integration:** Rapid advancements in healthcare technology require nurses to adapt to new systems, maintain digital literacy, and balance technology use with patient-centered care.
- **Advocacy and recognition:** Nurses may face challenges in advocating for their profession, securing fair compensation, and gaining recognition for their contributions to healthcare delivery and patient outcomes.

SUMMARY

In recent years, several trends have emerged in the field of nursing that are shaping the future of the profession. One significant trend is the increasing emphasis on technology in healthcare, leading to the adoption of electronic health records, telemedicine, and other digital tools to improve patient care and communication. Another trend is the growing focus on patient-centered care, which involves treating patients as partners in their own healthcare decisions and considering their individual preferences and needs. Additionally, there is a rising demand for nurses with specialized skills and knowledge in areas such as geriatrics, mental health, and community health, reflecting the changing demographics and healthcare needs of the population. The importance of interprofessional collaboration and teamwork in healthcare delivery is also a key trend, as nurses work closely with other healthcare professionals to provide holistic and coordinated care to patients. Finally, there is a growing recognition of the need for ongoing education and professional development in nursing, as new research, technologies, and best practices continue to evolve. By staying informed and adapting to these trends, nurses can enhance their practice and contribute to the advancement of healthcare delivery.

REVIEW QUESTIONS

Long Answer Question

1. Define trends in nursing and describe trends in nursing practices.

Short Answer Question

1. Discuss trends in nursing education.

Multiple Choice Questions

1. What is a key trend in nursing practices in the modern healthcare landscape?
   A. Increased focus on holistic care
   B. Decreased emphasis on evidence-based practice
   C. Limited use of technology in patient care
   D. Reduced importance of interdisciplinary collaboration

Ans: A. Increased focus on holistic care

Explanation: One of the key trends in nursing practices today is the shift towards providing holistic care, which considers the physical, emotional, social, and spiritual needs of patients. This approach recognizes the interconnectedness of various aspects of health and well-being, leading to more comprehensive and patient-centered care.

2. How has technology impacted nursing practices in recent years?
   A. Technology has had minimal impact on nursing care
   B. Technology has led to decreased efficiency in healthcare delivery
   C. Technology has improved communication and patient monitoring
   D. Technology has resulted in decreased patient safety

Ans: C. Technology has improved communication and patient monitoring

Explanation: Technology has significantly impacted nursing practices by enhancing communication among healthcare teams, enabling remote patient monitoring, facilitating electronic health records management, and improving the efficiency and accuracy of clinical processes.

Chapter 8

Telemedicine and Telenursing

> *"Education is not preparation for life; education is life itself."*
>
> —***John Dewey***

INTRODUCTION

Telemedicine is an emerging field in health science that results from the effective integration of information and communication technologies (ICT) with medical sciences. This innovative approach holds significant promise in addressing healthcare delivery challenges in rural and remote areas, as well as offering various applications in education, training, and health sector management. Telemedicine can range from simple interactions between two healthcare professionals discussing a patient's medical issues over the phone to more complex processes involving the transmission of electronic medical records, diagnostic tests like ECGs and radiological images, and conducting real-time interactive medical video conferences using IT-based hardware and software. These advancements in telemedicine also include video conferences facilitated by broadband telecommunication networks, whether through satellite or terrestrial connections.

TELEMEDICINE IN INDIA

One of the oldest known Telecardiology systems for Tele transmissions of ECGs was established in Gwalior, India in 1975 at GR Medical college. The first Ayurveda telemedicine center was established in India in 2007 by Dr Partap Chauhan, Director of Jiva Ayurveda.

Objectives

- To provide specialized medical advice.
- To monitor patient condition.

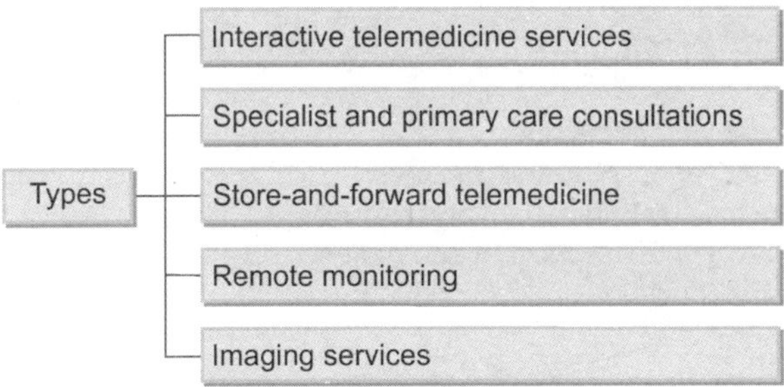

Fig. 8.1: Types of telemedicine.

- To guide other medical staff about treatment procedure.
- Share patient data among institutions for research purpose.

Types of Telemedicine

There are five types of telemedicine depicted in **Figure 8.1**.

Location

Can be located at any nonprime location away from the patient traffic near to communication system satellite.

Layout

- Reception
- Telemedicine conference hall
- Telemedicine library
- Cafeteria
- Restrooms

Staffing

- Head of the department
- Consultant
- Network manager
- Program manager
- Web developer
- Telemedicine technician
- Telephone attendant

Benefits of Telemedicine

- Window to expertise care
- Economic for hospital and patient
- Reduce the stress in patient and relatives
- Save travel time of specialist and patient
- Good for education and research purpose

Definition

- **Tele health:** It is the use of electronic information and telecommunications technologies to support long distance clinical health care, patient and professional health-related education, public health and health administration.
- **Telenursing:** It is a subset of telehealth in which technology is used to deliver nursing care and conduct nursing practice. It is specific to nursing as a profession. Telenursing is not a new mode of health care delivery rather it is an evolving mode of healthcare delivery that begun from the advent of telephone use in 1876. It refers to the use of telecommunications and information technology for providing nursing services in health care whenever a large physical distance exists between patient and nurse, or between any numbers of nurses. As a field it is part of telehealth, and has many points of contacts with other medical and nonmedical applications, such as telediagnosis, teleconsultation, telemonitoring, telecare, etc.

Types of Telenursing

- **Remote monitoring:** The nurse monitors the patient remotely from his/her house. Patients collect and transmit data to nurses; the nurse plans the intervention. Used for handling chronic diseases like heart disease, diabetes, asthma, etc.
- **Interactive telenursing services:** It involves series of interactive sessions with client via phone conversations and online communication. Used to obtain history, physical tests, psychiatric assessments, ophthalmology evaluation.
- **Store and forward telenursing:** Used to obtain medical images, audio or video data that can be forwarded to a nurse at a suitable time for evaluation offline. Areas utilized are dermatology, radiology and pathology.

- **Specialist and primary care consultations:** Patient sees a nurse over a live video connection or using diagnostic images/video along with patient data to a specialist for viewing later.
- **Imaging services:** Used in radiology, pathology and in cardiology.

Principles of Telenursing

- Augment existing heathcare services and expand the hospital services to remote areas.
- Enhance optimum and immediate access, thereby reducing chronic illness and hospitalizations.
- Improve and enhance the quality of care and maintain nursing standard and practices in a better way.
- Reduce the delivery of unnecessary health services by providing relevant information at real time.
- Protect confidentiality and security and consider patient right.

Functions of Telenursing

The functions of telenursing include providing the patient with informed consent, informing him/her of the choices, advocating technical innovations and systems that support safe, competent, and ethical care, complying with existing organizational policies and guidelines, providing the patient with the nurse's full name, qualifications, and registration.

Uses of Telenursing

- Telenursing was instituted as an effective mode for providing care to patients geographically distant from healthcare providers.
- Using telecommunications and information technology, nursing care is provided in remote areas.
- Nurses recognize the value of telecare and tele homecare as essential components of telenursing that give patients easy access to high-quality care and eliminate costs and difficulties associated with travel to healthcare facilities.
- Telenursing continues to grow as a valuable method for providing nursing care, especially in home health care.

Advantages and Disadvantages of Telenursing (Table 8.1)

Table 8.1: Advantages and disadvantages of telenursing.

Advantages	*Disadvantages*
To increases the access to healthcare services	Absence of direct hands and face to face direction
To reduce the cost	Technical difficulties
To reduce the visiting/waiting time/ unnecessary visit to hospital	Possibilities for health provider to step out of their scope of services
To provide immediate healthcare information to solve the problems	Increases the liability of risk
Medicare reimbursement	Inability to provide patients with information to make informed decisions
	Increase risk to security and confidentiality of clients with health information and records

Barriers of Telenursing

Barriers to telenursing include limitations in providing hands-on care and physical assessments, which can be crucial in certain medical situations. There may be challenges in establishing trust and rapport with patients through virtual interactions, potentially impacting the quality of care. Technical issues such as poor internet connectivity or equipment malfunctions can disrupt communication and care delivery. Additionally, concerns about data security and patient privacy in digital healthcare platforms may hinder the widespread adoption of telenursing. Regulatory and legal complexities, including varying state licensure requirements and insurance coverage for telehealth services, can also pose barriers to the implementation of telenursing practices. **Figure 8.2** depicts the barriers of telenursing.

- **Behavioral barriers**: It include resistance to telenursing — "fear that nurses are delegating tasks to machines."
- **Public barriers:** It include change management—understanding the capabilities and limitations of the technologies and applying them appropriately, lack of knowledge on information technology and usage among healthcare professionals and clients.
- **Financial barriers**: It include access to capital and responsibility issues such as who was going to pay for it and whether the

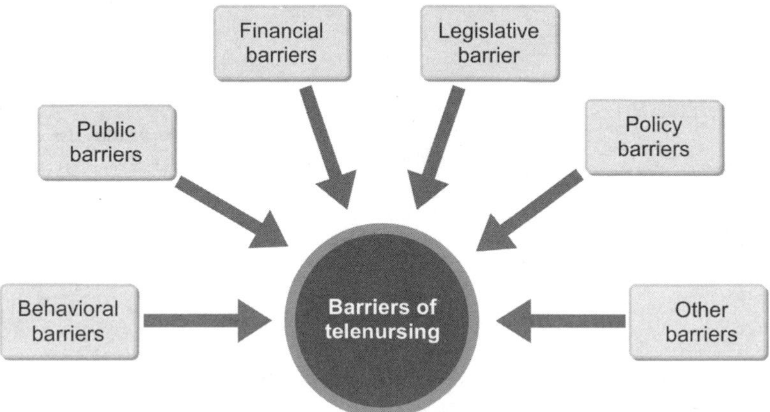

Fig. 8.2: Barriers of telenursing.

responsibility to sustain/add programs lay at the national, provincial, or regional level or was a combination of all of these.

- **Legislative barrier:** It include licensure, nursing, legal, ethical responsibilities, cross-jurisdictional issues, provincial/territorial response.
- **Policy barriers**: It include the absence of policies impacting telenursing adoption and lack of uniform standards provincially and nationally.
- **Other barriers**: They are the potential for fraud and abuse, privacy concerns, secure access, and consent management. The type required, who should obtain, the secondary use of data, for example, research.

Applications

There are three application of telenursing which is depicted in **Figure 8.3**.

- **Home care:** One of the most distinctive telenursing applications is home care. For example, patients who are immobilized, or live in remote or difficult to reach places, citizens who have chronic ailments, such as chronic obstructive pulmonary disease, diabetes, congestive heart disease, or debilitating diseases, such as neural degenerative diseases (Parkinson's disease, Alzheimer's disease or ALS), may stay at home and be "visited" and assisted regularly by a nurse via videoconferencing, internet or videophone. Other

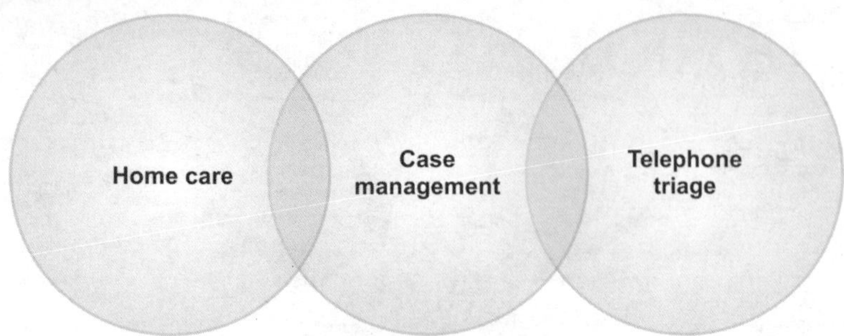

Fig. 8.3: Application of telenursing.

applications of home care are the care of patients in immediate postsurgical situations, the care of wounds, ostomies or disabled individuals. In normal home health care, one nurse is able to visit up to 5–7 patients per day. Using telenursing, one nurse can "visit" 12–16 patients in the same amount of time.

- **Case management:** A common application of telenursing is also used by call centers operated by managed care organizations, which are staffed by registered nurses who act as case managers or perform patient triage, information and counseling as a means of regulating patient access and flow and decrease the use of emergency rooms.
- **Telephone triage:** It refers to symptom or clinically based calls. Clinicians perform symptom assessment by asking detailed questions about the patient's illness or injury. The clinician's task is to estimate and/or rule out urgent symptoms. They may use pattern recognition and other problem-solving process as well. Clinicians may utilize guidelines, in paper or electronic format, to determine how urgent the symptoms are. Telephone triage requires clinicians to determine if the symptoms are life-threatening, emergency, urgent, acute or non-acute. It may involve educating and advising clients, and making safe, effective, and appropriate dispositions—all by telephone. Telephone triage takes place in settings as diverse as emergency rooms, ambulance services, large call centers, physician offices, clinics, student health centers and hospices.

Legal, Ethical and Regulatory Issues

- Telenursing is fraught with legal, ethical and regulatory issues, as it happens with telehealth as a whole.

- In many countries, interstate and intercountry practice of telenursing is forbidden (the attending nurse must have a license both in their state/country of residence and in the state/country where the patient receiving telecare is located).
- The Nurse Licensure Compact helps resolve some of these jurisdiction issues.
- Legal issues such as accountability and malpractice, etc., are also still largely unsolved and difficult to address.
- Ethical issues include maintaining autonomy, maintaining a patients integrity as well as preventing harm to a patient.
- In addition, there are many considerations related to patient confidentiality and safety of clinical data.
- Accountability for practice, security, privacy, and confidentiality, providing informed consent, and liability protection are some of the legal, ethical, and regulatory issues in telenursing. In India Anna University, Apollo Telemedicine Networking Foundation provides a certificate course, School of Telemedicine and Biomedical Informatics, National Institute of Health and Family Welfare, and Rad Gurukul provide training in telenursing.

Implications of Telenursing

For the Patients

- Monitoring vital signs
- Provide opportunities for early intervention
- Reduce the number of visits to the doctors or emergency department
- Provides patient education
- Removes geographic and sometimes financial barriers
- Improve accessibility to specialists

For the Providers

- Competencies and scope of practices
- Local accountability
- Client safety
- Client security, confidentiality and privacy
- Informed content obtained
- Involved client decision making
- Professional practice environment

For the Healthcare System

- Initial expenses at first but as health improves, the system will save money.
- Decreased number of in hospital days for patients with chronic illness who have access to supportive telehealth.
- Decreases the number of in-hospital days.
- Reduce the required number of staff (nursing in particular).
- Removes the barriers of time and distance.
- Proper training and administration support is a vital responsibility for the system.

SUMMARY

Telenursing is a very important for our country; it needs to be implemented because by using telenursing, nurses will be able to assess patient conditions, provide the best nursing care, and evaluate the effectiveness of nursing care from distant locations. Telenursing may also be used for the purpose of follow-up of the client. Telenursing also helps the patient to get nursing care at their homes and communities where the facilities are not developed. It also reduces the traveling for both the patient and the nurse. In short, telenursing may be used for the primary, secondary, and tertiary management of clients.

REVIEW QUESTIONS

Long Answer Question

1. Define telenursing, its advantages and disadvantages and applications in nursing.

Short Answer Questions

1. Explain implications of telenursing.
2. Enlist the type of telemedicine.

Multiple Choice Questions

1. Which of the following is a benefit of telenursing?
   A. Increased face-to-face interaction with patients
   B. Limited access to healthcare services
   C. Improved access to healthcare in remote areas
   D. Decreased use of technology in healthcare

Ans: C. Improved access to healthcare in remote areas

Explanation: Telenursing helps improve access to healthcare services in remote or underserved areas by allowing patients to receive care and consultations from nurses and healthcare providers through telecommunication technologies.

2. What is an essential skill for tele nurses?
   A. Proficiency in traditional paper charting
   B. Ability to communicate effectively through technology
   C. Limited knowledge of medical terminology
   D. Lack of adaptability to new technologies

Ans: B. Ability to communicate effectively through technology

Explanation: Telenurses need to have strong communication skills to effectively interact with patients, colleagues, and healthcare providers through various technological platforms used in telenursing.

3. Which of the following is a potential challenge of telenursing?
   A. Limited access to healthcare services
   B. Decreased patient satisfaction
   C. Difficulty in establishing rapport with patients
   D. Increased healthcare costs

Ans: C. Difficulty in establishing rapport with patients

Explanation: One of the challenges of telenursing is the potential difficulty in establishing a strong rapport and connection with patients compared to in-person interactions. Telenurses need to find ways to build trust and communication effectively through technology.

4. How can telenursing benefit patients with chronic conditions?
   A. By providing immediate emergency care
   B. By reducing the need for regular follow-up appointments
   C. By offering continuous monitoring and support
   D. By limiting access to specialized healthcare services

Ans: C. By offering continuous monitoring and support

Explanation: Telenursing can benefit patients with chronic conditions by providing continuous monitoring, support, and education remotely, helping them manage their conditions more effectively and improving their overall health outcomes.

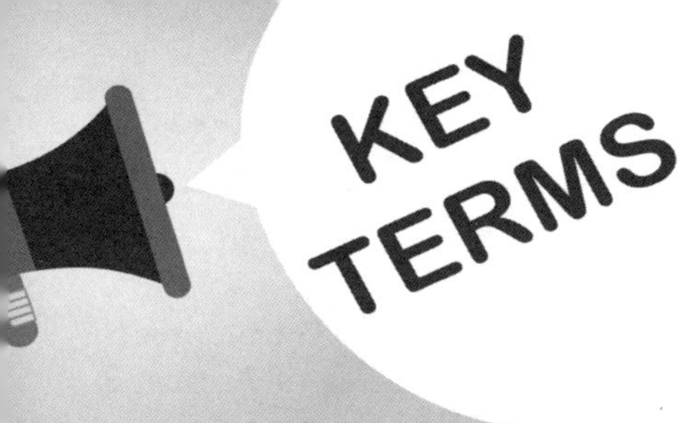

- **Active euthanasia:** The ending of another person's life by an aggressive method to end suffering.
- **American civil war:** A conflict fought in the United States from 1861 to 1865, during which nursing gained recognition and importance through the efforts of figures like Clara Barton.
- **Assault:** A deliberate act wherein one person threatens to harm another without consent and the victim feels the attacker has the ability to carry out the threat.
- **Basic nursing care:** Care that can be performed following a defined nursing procedure with minimal modification in which the responses of the patient to the nursing care are predictable.
- **Board of nursing:** The state-specific licensing and regulatory body that sets the standards for safe nursing care, decides the scope of practice for nurses within its jurisdiction, and issues licenses to qualified candidates.
- **Chain of command:** A hierarchy of reporting relationships in an agency that establishes accountability and lays outlines of authority and decision-making power.
- **Crimean war:** A conflict fought from 1853 to 1856, during which Florence Nightingale and a team of nurses made significant contributions to healthcare and established nursing as a respected profession.
- **Code of ethics:** A code that applies normative, moral guidance for nurses in terms of what they ought to do, be, and seek. A code of ethics makes the primary obligations, values, and ideals of a profession explicit.
- **Dysphagia:** Impaired swallowing.
- **Empathy:** Intellectual and emotional awareness and understanding of another person's thoughts behaviors and feelings.
- **Ethical principle:** An ethical principle is a general guide, basic truth, or assumption that can be used with clinical judgment to determine a course of action. Four common ethical principles are

beneficence (do good), nonmaleficence (do no harm), autonomy (control by the individual), and justice (fairness).

- **Evidence-based practice:** A lifelong problem-solving approach that integrates the best evidence from well-designed research studies and evidence-based theories; clinical expertise and evidence from assessment of the health consumer's history and condition, as well as healthcare resources; and patient, family, group, community, and population preferences and values.
- **Geriatric nurse:** It is a specialized healthcare professional who focuses on providing comprehensive nursing care to elderly individuals. Also known as gerontological nurses or elderly care nurses, they have specialized knowledge and skills to address the unique healthcare needs and challenges associated with aging. Geriatric nurses work in various healthcare settings, including hospitals, long-term care facilities, rehabilitation centers, and community health agencies.
- **Holistic nursing:** An approach to nursing that considers the whole person—body, mind, and spirit—emphasizing the interconnectedness of these aspects for comprehensive healthcare.
- **International Council of Nurses (ICN):** A global organization representing nurses worldwide, working to advance nursing and healthcare standards on an international level.
- **Infection control:** Practices and protocols to prevent the spread of infections in healthcare settings.
- **Informed consent:** The legal and ethical requirement that no significant medical procedure can be performed until the competent patient has been informed of the nature of the procedure, risks and alternatives, as well as the prognosis if the procedure is not done. The patient must freely and voluntarily agree to have the procedure done.
- **Licensed practical nurse/vocational nurse (LPN/LVN):** An individual who has completed a state-approved practical or vocational nursing program, passed the NCLEX-PN examination, and is licensed by their state Board of Nursing to provide patient care.
- **Mental health nursing:** A specialized field focusing on the care and treatment of individuals with mental health disorders, evolving over time to address the unique needs of this patient population.

- **Midwifery:** The practice of assisting women during childbirth, with a long history that predates modern nursing and continues to be a significant aspect of healthcare.
- **Nightingale pledge**: A modified version of the Hippocratic Oath, taken by nurses upon graduation, expressing their commitment to ethical nursing practice.
- **Nursing:** Nursing integrates the art and science of caring and focused on the protection, promotion, and optimization of health and human functioning; prevention of illness and injury; facilitation of healing; and alleviation of suffering through compassionate presence. Nursing is the diagnosis and treatment of human responses and advocacy in the care of individuals, families, groups, communities, and populations in recognition of the connection of all humanity.
- **Nursing theories:** Frameworks and conceptual models developed by nurse theorists to guide and explain nursing practice, such as those by Virginia Henderson, Dorothea Orem, and Jean Watson.
- **Nurse Practice Act (NPA):** Legislation enacted by each state that establishes regulations for nursing practice within that state by defining the requirements for licensure, as well as the scope of nursing practice.
- **Nurse Practitioner (NP):** A highly trained and specialized nurse with advanced education and clinical training, often able to diagnose and treat medical conditions independently.
- **Oncology:** Study of cancer
- **OR:** Operating room
- **Patient confidentiality:** Keeping your patient's protected health information (PHI) protected and known only by those healthcare team members directly providing care for the patient.
- **Primary care:** Care that is provided to patients to promote wellness and prevent disease from occurring. This includes health promotion, education, protection (such as immunizations), early disease screening, and environmental considerations.
- **Profession:** A profession is an occupation with moral principles that are devoted to the human and social welfare. The service is based on specialized knowledge and skill developed in a scientific and learned manner.
- **Professional conduct:** Professional conduct is behaving with a real sense of dignity and respect for the service given for the patient and for theses with which one works.

- **Protocol:** A precise and detailed written plan for a regimen of therapy.
- **Provider:** A physician, podiatrist, dentist, optometrist, or advanced practice nurse provider.
- **Public health nursing:** A field of nursing focused on promoting and protecting the health of communities and populations, often involving outreach and preventive healthcare measures.
- **Quality:** The degree to which nursing services for healthcare consumers, families, groups, communities, and populations increase the likelihood of desirable outcomes and are consistent with evolving nursing knowledge.
- **Red cross:** An international humanitarian organization founded by Henry Dunant and Clara Barton, providing aid and relief in times of war and disaster.
- **Registered nurse (RN):** An individual who has graduated from a state-approved school of nursing, passed the NCLEX-RN examination, and is licensed by a state board of nursing to provide patient care.
- **Safety culture:** A culture established within healthcare agencies that empowers nurses, nursing students, and other staff members to speak up about risks to patients and to report errors and near misses, all of which drive improvement in patient care and reduce the incident of patient harm.
- **Scope of practice:** Services that a qualified health professional is deemed competent to perform and permitted to undertake—in keeping with the terms of their professional license.
- **Secondary care:** Care that occurs when a person has contracted an illness or injury and is in need of medical care.
- **Tertiary care:** A type of care that deals with the long-term effects from chronic illness or condition, with the purpose to restore physical and mental function that may have been lost. The goal is to achieve the highest level of functioning possible with this chronic illness.
- **Travel nurse:** A nurse who works for short periods of time with different healthcare facilities.
- **Values:** Values are persistent convictions or attitudes regarding the significance of individuals, concepts, or behaviors. They hold significance as they shape decisions and behaviors, including the ethical decision-making process of nurses.
- **World Health Organization (WHO):** A global organization that plays a key role in shaping international health policies and standards, promoting nursing as an integral part of health care.

Index

Page numbers followed by *f* refer to figure and *t* refer to table

A

Advocacy 40, 45, 71, 82
Alzheimer's disease 89
Ambiguity, acceptance of 71
American Civil War 95
Anuraktha 26
Assault 95
Autonomy 69
Auxiliary nurse midwives 49, 51

B

Basic nursing
  care 95
  principles 42
Behavioral barriers 88
Beneficence 69
Bhore committee 51
Burnout 45, 82

C

Care, nature of 75
Civilian nursing 15, 28
Clear communication 71
Collaboration 41
Communication technologies 84
Community
  health
    nurse 16, 32
    service, nursing personnel in 39
  nursing 46
Confidentiality 70
Crimean War 95
Cross roads, nursing of 57

D

Dais 16
Daksha 25
Diversity 45
Duty pattern 77
Dysphagia 95

E

Education 46
  mode of 78
Eligibility criteria 55
Empathy 95
Employment opportunities, expansion of 78
Ethical dilemmas 45, 70, 82
Ethical issues 70, 90
Ethical principles 68, 68*f*, 95
Ethics, code of 65, 66*f*, 95
Euthanasia, active 95
Evidence-based practice 78, 96
Excellence 40

F

Fidelity 69
Financial barriers 88
Florence Nightingale 19, 20*f*
  contributions of 19
Framework application 72

G

General nursing 52
Geriatric nurse 96
Global health 78
  challenges 80
Global opportunities 47

H

Healthcare 5
  policy and legislation 79
  system 92
  technology, advancement in 79
Holistic nursing 96
Home care 89

I

Imaging services 87
Inclusion 45

Indian Nursing Council 51, 59
Industrial nurse 32
Infection control 96
Information technology 84
  advancement in 76
Informed consent 96
Integrity 40
Interactive telenursing services 86
International Council of Nurses 62, 96
International influence 21
Interprofessional collaboration 76, 80

J

Justice 69

K

Kartar Singh Committee 50, 51

L

Lady health visitors 50, 51
Legal awareness 72
Legal issues 90
Legislative barrier 89
Licensed practical nurse 96

M

Marital status criteria 77
Maternal and child health 50
Mental health 82
  nursing 96
Mentally ill, special care of 14
Midwifery 52, 97
Military nursing 27, 32
  history of 14
Missionary nursing 16, 28
Modern nursing, founder of 20
Moral distress 70
Mudaliar Committee 50, 51

N

Nightingale pledge 97
Nonmaleficence 69
Nurse 37, 67
  administrators leadership behavior 76
  assignment of 77
  functions of 43, 44*f*, 71
  practice act 61, 97
  practitioner 97
    programs 55
    role of 56, 76
  preparation 77
  role of 3, 4, 43, 44*f*, 71, 75
  shortage of 45
Nursing 1, 23-27, 37, 97
  agency 75
  ancient history of 23
  and Midwifery Council 59
  audit 58
  board of 95
  care
    delivery, mode of 75
    focus on 75
    type of 75
  concept of 37
  current trends in 59
  education 21, 29, 49
    development of 49
    evolution of 49
    nursing personnel in 39
    outline of 57
    trends in 79, 80*f*
  ethical aspects of 65
  factors affecting trends in 79
  historical development in 1
  history of 2
  institutions, number of 77
  issues in 81, 81*f*
  leadership 32
  legacy in 21
  milestones of 30
  objectives of 41
  philosophy of 37
  practice
    nature of 38, 38*t*
    scope of 38, 38*t*
    trends in 75
  profession 45
    types of 38
  program 38
    type of 77
  research in 58
  scope of 31, 45
  service
    abroad 32
    administrative positions 32
  shortages 80, 82
  superintendent 32
  teaching in 32
  theories 97
  trends in 74
  type of 75

O

Oncology 97

P

Parkinson's disease 89
Patient-centered care 80

Policy 45
  barriers 89
Post basic certificate courses 53
Practice, scope of 45, 82, 98
Profession 35, 97
  characteristics of 36
Professional conduct 97
Professional development 45, 82
  opportunities 80
Professional nurse, qualities of 42, 43*f*
Public health 46
  advocacy for 21
  nurses 51, 98

R

Recognition 72, 82
Red cross 98
Registered nurse 98
Regulatory issues 90
Research 46
Resources, lack of 82
Rights 69

S

Safety 41
  culture 98
Sanitary reforms 21
Self-awareness 71
Shrivastav Committee 50, 51
State Nursing Councils 60
Stress 45
Systematic problem-solving 71

T

Technology integration 82
Telehealth 86
Telemedicine 84
  benefits of 86
  types of 85
Telenursing 84, 86
  advantages of 88, 88*t*
  application of 90*f*
  barriers of 88, 89*f*
  disadvantages of 88, 88*t*
  functions of 87
  implications of 91
  principles of 87
  types of 86
  uses of 87
Telephone triage 90
Trained Nurses Association of India 61

V

Vocational nurse 96

W

Workforce diversity 82
Workplace violence 45, 82
World Health Organization 98